Special Praise for
Loving Our Addicted Daughters Back to Life

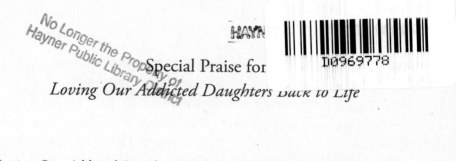

"*Loving Our Addicted Daughters Back to Life* is a heartbreaking and also heartwarming testament to the need to understand and address addiction as a preventable and treatable disease. As Linda Dahl eloquently demonstrates, countless families are not aware of the risk factors for this disease, how it may affect girls and women differently, or what to do if they have to face it. Instead, they are left to sift through a confusing array of providers rarely offering treatment known to be effective, and to blame themselves for relapses resulting from inadequate treatment or the disease itself. *Loving Our Addicted Daughters Back to Life* is an important resource for families, especially families with daughters. It is a message of hope—that addiction can be prevented and treated effectively and that people with the disease can learn to manage it and live healthy, productive lives."

—Susan E. Foster, Executive Director, ABAM Foundation's National
Center for Physician Training in Addiction Medicine, and principal
investigator for *Women Under the Influence*, the National Center on
Addiction and Substance Abuse (CASA) at Columbia University

"This is a very valuable and important book. Linda Dahl has written a touching and compassionate guide for those who are seeking addiction treatment for their daughters. She has clearly outlined the pain that mothers experience, as well as the need for and importance of specialized services for women and girls. As I think of the mothers who have called me over the years seeking advice about how to help their daughters, I wish I had had this resource to recommend. Any mother who is struggling to help her daughter will find *Loving Our Addicted Daughters* to be a gift."

—Stephanie S. Covington, PhD, psychotherapist and
author of *A Woman's Way through the Twelve Steps*

"*Loving Our Addicted Daughters Back to Life* is a significant contribution to the concerns around women and addiction. While validating the gut-wrenching pain of a mother with an addicted daughter, the book is offset with hopeful practical tips on discerning a chemical problem, finding help, as well as sensitive suggestions for greater understanding and hope. A timely reading with a balance of anecdote and research."

—Brenda J. Iliff, former Director of Hazelden Women's
Recovery Center and author of *A Woman's Guide to Recovery*

"*Loving Our Addicted Daughters Back to Life* brings hope to parents who have daughters struggling with addiction. Linda Dahl articulately combines her personal journey with some of the latest gender-specific addiction treatment research. This easy-to-follow guide provides parents with practical tools and resources, including a much-needed comparative listing of treatment centers."

—Michael Gurian, co-founder of the Gurian
Institute and author of *The Wonder of Girls*

Loving
Our Addicted
Daughters
Back to Life

Loving
Our Addicted
Daughters
Back to Life

A Guidebook for Parents

LINDA DAHL

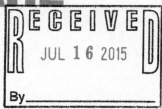
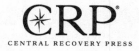

CRP®

CENTRAL RECOVERY PRESS

Las Vegas

Central Recovery Press (CRP) is committed to publishing exceptional materials addressing addiction treatment, recovery, and behavioral healthcare topics, including original and quality books, audio/visual communications, and web-based new media. Through a diverse selection of titles, we seek to contribute a broad range of unique resources for professionals, recovering individuals and their families, and the general public.

For more information, visit www.centralrecoverypress.com.

Publisher: Central Recovery Press
3321 N. Buffalo Drive
Las Vegas, NV 89129

20 19 18 17 16 15   1 2 3 4 5

ISBN: 978-1-937612-85-6 (paper)
978-1-937612-86-3 (e-book)

Author photo by Duanne Shinkle-Simon. Used with permission.

Step One of the Twelve Step Program of Alcoholics Anonymous on page 85 reprinted by permission of AA World Services, Inc. All rights reserved.

Quote from *Alcoholics Anonymous*, 4th ed., page 33, reprinted on page 85 with permission of AA World Services, Inc. All rights reserved.

Publisher's Note: This book contains general information about addiction, addiction recovery, and related matters. The information is not medical advice, and should not be treated as such. Central Recovery Press makes no representations or warranties in relation to the information in this book. If you have any specific questions about any medical matter discussed in this book, you should consult your doctor or other professional healthcare provider. This book is not an alternative to medical advice from your doctor or other professional healthcare provider.

Our books represent the experiences and opinions of their authors only. Every effort has been made to ensure that events, institutions, and statistics presented in our books as facts are accurate and up-to-date. To protect their privacy, the names of some of the people, places, and institutions in this book may have been changed.

Cover design and interior design and layout by Deb Tremper, Six Penny Graphics.

This book is for parents and loved ones who know a
young woman who is using alcohol or other drugs.
May it guide you to love her, and yourself, back to health.

Table of Contents

Acknowledgments

My deep appreciation goes out to the families and young women who shared their stories in these pages. Also to the many dedicated professionals for their passion to impart knowledge that improves the odds for recovery from addiction for young women. To the parents of children with a substance use disorder who are committed to helping other such families. To the memory of Susan Zeckendorf, my longtime agent and dear friend. To Martha, my wonderful sponsor and friend: we were young alcoholics and drug users who took the help offered to us to recover from addiction and in four decades, we have never looked back. To my beloved daughter "Kim" (whose name, like that of all those who have shared their personal stories, has been changed to protect her privacy). You fought for your life, emerging from the depths of active addiction to become a vibrant example of recovery today. Finally, to the many young women and men and the parents I've met who are working toward recovery and to those I haven't yet met. You are living proof there is hope for the future.

"Girls and young women use cigarettes, alcohol and other drugs for different reasons than boys and young men. [They] are more vulnerable than boys to substance abuse and addiction and its consequences."

—The National Center on Addiction and Substance Abuse at Columbia University (CASAColumbia)

Introduction

An eminent physician who has worked for decades with young people suffering from addiction describes the drug crisis today in words that should shock and awe all of us: "We are experiencing the worst drug addiction epidemic in United States history."[1]

Whether it's called substance use, risky use, drug dependence, substance abuse, substance use disorder, substance use disease, addiction, or alcoholism, taking mood-changing, mind-altering chemicals that may become habit-forming can at any point be harmful to the user. The label may carry shades of different meanings, but it's the destructive illness that matters. Experimenting with alcohol and/or other drugs will lead only some to heartbreak and addiction, but, like in Russian roulette, nobody knows when the gun will fire.

The statistics about people suffering from the effects of addiction to alcohol and/or a raft of other drugs, especially opiates and, above all, heroin, are so chilling you would think we'd all be out marching in the streets as people did about HIV/AIDS. To cite just one statistic: heroin deaths were up 39 percent in 2013 from the previous year.[2] You'd think we'd be besieging our legislators en masse for more treatments that work, prevention strategies that our kids can actually relate to, and vaccines to halt the horrors of addiction. But before we get to that, let me pose a question: What parent wants to believe they have raised a drug addict or alcoholic before the reality of it explodes in his or her face? None who I have met or read about during the years I spent researching this book. And that includes me, the mother of a daughter who was addicted from her teens into her twenties. Many seem to think it's a problem that won't ever touch their kids (that would be me). Take a recent nationwide survey of a diverse group of some 2,500 parents, which found most parents of twelve- to twenty-four-year-olds say they're not concerned about their kids' possible use. About 80 percent of these parents think they would know how to read the signs (if, God forbid, their child somehow started experimenting), but were only able to identify two out of thirty-eight possible indications of kids' using.[3] Even scarier are the results from a survey of middle-schoolers from my own community that reports the majority of kids don't think their parents would mind if they used drugs.

Reality comes crashing down when good, smart, nice young people use drugs.

If you've picked up this book out of concern for your child or a loved one's possible addiction, you're not alone: Risky substance use is being called the leading public healthcare problem for young people in America.[4] Addiction originates before the age of twenty-one in 96.5 percent of cases.[5] The most current data show 1.3 million Americans ages twelve to seventeen—that's 5.2 percent of adolescents—had a substance use disorder in 2013, meaning an alcohol or drug dependence requiring treatment. Nearly another million teens were illicit drug users who did not meet the criteria for dependence, and 1.6 million reported recent binge drinking (there is no official breakdown for young adults older than seventeen).[6]

Let's turn now to our daughters, our nieces, our granddaughters, and children of friends and neighbors. Again, girls are more likely than boys to intentionally abuse prescription drugs to get high. Among twelve- to seventeen-year-olds, girls are more likely than boys to abuse prescription drugs, pain relievers, tranquilizers, and stimulants.[7] As I write this, girls and young women are the fastest-growing group of addicts in the country. *Yes, you read that right.* The government estimates 58 percent of the 7,800 people over the age of twelve who tried an illicit drug for the first time in 2013 were females.[8] Approximately 8.6 million women are reported to be addicted: nearly 6 million women to alcohol and 2.6 million to other drugs.[9]

Those of us who have faced the searingly painful reality of a young woman's risky use or dependence agonize over why. Why are so many girls and young women with so much promise using and abusing substances that are so harmful to their health? The reasons are both complex and enlightening. Among them: risky (or binge) drinking and drug use, including opiates (painkillers obtained legally or illegally, and heroin) have become de-stigmatized for many kids of this generation. Also, there is a sense of entitlement and empowerment connected to drinking and drugging for some young women today that is intimately and insidiously bound up with youth culture and advertising. Are we aware of the rise in binge drinking? It has increased to the point that it now affects about 30 percent of high school students and up to 60 percent in many colleges.[10] Added to the mix may be marijuana, cocaine, Ecstasy, methamphetamine, "designer" drugs, and many others I will describe in later chapters. Another reason girls turn to substances is that with the onset of puberty they often experience depression, eating and body image disorders, and/or anxiety at a significantly higher rate than their male peers—who, on the other hand, have higher rates of autism and attention deficit disorder.[11] Finally, and crucially, young women's substance use is often fueled by the experience of abuse and/or trauma. It happens far more often than we like to think. Young women are very good at keeping secrets.

Above all, what's driving our current worst-ever drug epidemic for young people is the widespread availability of prescription painkillers and heroin. Opiates have acquired a reputation for giving the user the best feeling in the world ever, a perfect way to resolve the stress and social anxieties that go along with being a teenager. And because of their fast-acting, highly addictive nature, opiates are causing more and more kids to become dependent, with disastrous consequences. *Opiates* are derived from naturally-occurring alkaloids in the opium poppy. In contrast, *opioids* are synthetic, produced in the laboratory (although the effects of opiates and opioids are virtually identical). These drugs induce feelings of euphoria and drastically reduce the perception of pain. Because of the way they are processed in the brain they are wickedly quick to create a need for more in the user. Often, the new user will start off taking pills, graduate to sniffing ground-up powdered pills, and in many cases go on to inject it. And since a main culprit—the prescription opioid painkiller Oxycontin— has been made tamper-proof, more and more kids are turning to a more available and cheaper opiate: heroin. It floods the country, trucked in from Mexico, and is much cheaper than prescription pain pills—and potent. As with other "street drugs," there is no way for the user to ascertain the strength of a given batch of heroin nor its adulteration with other substances (such as the potent painkiller fentanyl), making it even more dangerous. Another hazard stems from adolescent users' tendency to mix drugs, such as taking opiates together with Xanax or alcohol.

Women are especially at risk of becoming addicted to opiates/opioids. As one expert explains, women "accelerate to injecting drugs at a faster rate than men . . . develop[ing] substance disorders in less time than men. . . . Women of all ages suffer greater physical, psychological, and social consequences."[12] In plain language, females get sicker on chemicals faster than males. I hammer away at this point because while the addiction rate is climbing among young women, they continue to be—as they have been historically—under-diagnosed, misdiagnosed, and/or not treated appropriately.

This book focuses on what we need to do to effectively help them, as well as ourselves. You will find the best prevention tools: knowledge about effective means of intervening and finding good treatment, and many new discoveries and techniques that specifically aid female addicts but are still not widely known or properly implemented. I will provide you with practical, time-tested ways of regaining your own well-being while dealing with an addicted daughter. In fact, taking care of ourselves may be the most important thing we parents can do!

There is clearly an urgent need for more effective prevention and treatment for everyone, from primary school on up. This includes taking into account important differences in the way girls and boys mature and handle stress. Young men and women who become addicted share many symptoms and have similar needs to recover, but there are also important differences between the genders that can be critical for proper diagnosis and treatment. For example, groundbreaking research in the study of hormonal fluctuations has opened up promising new therapies to help women avoid relapse as their hormones surge during their menstrual cycle. Other new findings targeting the specific needs of young women in science, psychology, and sociology are brought together for the first time in later chapters.

If you are a parent or caregiver who suspects or knows your daughter or young woman you care about is using addictive substances, I know you just want it to stop. You want it to go away. You want your daughter back. I know because I've been there. Faced with feelings of failure, fear, betrayal, anger, and shame, how can we choose or help her to choose the best action to take? We are in a serious, unending crisis, because dealing with addiction is like being on a battlefield. In such a state of mind, how do we evaluate and find effective treatment? Since every rehabilitation center's website claims to be effective, how do we know what works?

While this book touches on the urgent needs of substance users who are pregnant or mothers, those with varied cultural, racial, or ethnic needs, as well as our young sons, the main focus will be on the legion of single girls and young women at risk. Some are hopeful that we as a country are at a turning point in terms of treating addiction as a medical and often a psychiatric disorder and I share their yearning that the best and latest science-based techniques will become widespread. But those of us who are affected by the disease of addiction *now* can't wait.

What you will find in these pages:

- Best evidence-based approaches and new scientific research findings about young women and addiction
- Practical tips on how to assess a potential or actual addiction
- How to take meaningful preventive actions
- What kind of conversation works with your daughter
- The best way to assess her situation
- How to find and finance the most effective treatment
- The ways young women and men manifest signs of addiction differently
- How addiction affects women specifically
- Why underlying or accompanying mental health issues must be identified and treated concurrently in young women
- How differing evidence-based approaches in treatment can be crucial to both genders

- How triggers for relapse can be part of recovery and how they differ for women
- Tools and resources to help you and your family regain vitality and a fuller life

Treatment is increasingly being tailored to be effective for our young women today. Much has been learned in recent years to enhance their treatment, and today as never before parents have a key role to play in our children's lives when it comes to addiction and recovery.

Brenda's Story

More than one in four high school girls binge drink (five or more drinks on one occasion), and are five times more likely to have sex—and a third less likely to use protection—than girls who don't drink.[13]

Brenda, a bright, attractive young woman of twenty-two, is the oldest of three children in a stable family with two parents. She was raised in a lovely town in Southern California which, like so many suburban towns today, has a lot of alcohol and other drug problems among its young people. Her mother Abby tells their story.

"Brenda was a bright, beautiful, gifted child who got a lot of attention for her looks from an early age. Brenda seemed to have it all. She excelled in school and took up dance in pre-school. But by the time she was in junior high, in the eighth grade, she was already drinking. I didn't know, but there were signs. She quit dancing, she took up with different friends, and some of the parents weren't being responsible—they covered for her. When she got her driver's license she was driving drunk. She wouldn't come home. And she had an abusive boyfriend who terrified her—really creepy, horrible. He threatened the family. Her self-esteem tanked, and she started hanging out with the bottom-feeders. She became defiant about anything and would freak out in a second. I became afraid of her anger. I didn't want to upset her but I became her target. I stopped functioning and worried about her every second. I lost a lot of weight, couldn't sleep, and I was neglecting the family. Her dad just checked out; he was angry and couldn't handle it.

"We tried counseling, therapists. They knew she was drinking, involved in risky behavior, but she snowed them. I realized I was in way over my head, and I had to come to terms with the reality. I thought codependency was being a mom, but I had to get real. And Brenda showed some signs that she knew what she was doing. She would leave these little 'I'm sorry' notes. She would sleep in Mom's bed. I'm telling my husband her behavior's not normal and I start looking for alternatives. The turning point for him was one night when she was drunk and was trying to get in the car and leave. We're in the garage trying to stop her and her dad, who's a big guy, had to pin her down. She was wild and she banged her head on the concrete floor. We called the cops and they took her to the hospital, where she was horrible, just violent. When she came home, we said, 'You have one more chance.' Brenda walked out. We realized she was going to kill herself.

"Two people had recommended a facility in Utah to us. We pulled her out of high school in March of her junior year. We knew nothing about the school in Utah except that it had been recommended. She flew out and we couldn't see her for sixty days. It was a thirteen-month program where she would get her high school diploma, counseling, and treatment. And it was not cheap. We used her college fund to pay for it and borrowed on credit cards. It was money well spent. Our youngest daughter was so much younger that she was not involved and was okay. But our son would stay away from us, stay with friends. He started sobbing, saying it was his fault after Brenda went away. He was a straight arrow, never in trouble. He began having problems academically and I was worried about him, but he became a stellar athlete. Still, at the time he was so angry at her.

"It was a tough place in Utah that took in a variety of troubled kids and put them in groups according to their problem. There are lawsuits today by former students. But the timing was right for Brenda and her counselor was wonderful with her. After sixty days, we went out for weekends. When we visited, I got tense and had a hard time. I sobbed. I thought at first she was a wayward kid, I didn't think she was an alcoholic. We hoped she would just grow of it. But Brenda said, 'Mom, I'm an alcoholic.' I was so sad about the stigma. Alcoholism runs on both sides of our family and her dad is a situational drinker. But I kept talking to her counselor—who was wonderful—once a week. And then there was a required weekend intensive seminar for families. There were about a hundred parents with a facilitator. The seminar made me really uncomfortable. It opened my eyes and changed me. I had been horrified by her behavior, but I learned it was not a reflection on me, even though I felt it was. I would hang on to stuff. I learned there that Brenda needed to hear us say, 'We forgive you. But you need to forgive yourself so you can move forward.' It was powerful for us parents.

"There was no access to the outside world at the center, it was a locked-down facility that was closely supervised. It was co-ed, but they were kept separate. To re-integrate into the outside world, Brenda had to work out a life contract with the family, which we all signed, in which she gradually earned more freedom. Her counselor told us all, 'I *guarantee* success if you graduate the life contract.' It was a six-month process, then she went away to college. There, she did get together with a second abusive boyfriend. He was not welcome at our home. It took her a year to let go of him. And she didn't want to do the twelve-step program thing at first. She went to a women's meeting and wouldn't open up. But later she got into it and now she has a really good sponsor. And we're supportive. Parents need to be supportive of twelve-step programs for their kids.

"Now Brenda has been in recovery for five years. She's graduated from college and is going to get her master's. She wants to work with junior high school students to educate them about the dangers of alcohol and other drug abuse. When I talk to her now, she's loving her recovery and knows she wouldn't be alive today without it.

"We know other parents, wonderful families, who have lost their children to addiction. What I tell other parents is: Don't ignore it. Denial gets out of hand. Nip it early or it can be too late. Many parents aren't holding their kids accountable. They think they are 'protecting' their kids. But you have to pull the trigger. Don't be afraid of their anger. Also, parents are often divorced. But they have to be on the same page about this. You have to be uncomfortable enough to change. And it's worth all of it."

Notes on the Introduction

1. Andrew Kolodny, Chief Medical Officer of Phoenix House, a long-established rehabilitation center, and President of Physicians for Responsible Opioid Prescribing (PROP), in a Statement for the Record to Senator Levin and Senator Hatch titled "Buprenorphine in the Treatment of Opioid Addiction: Successes and the Impediments to Expanded Access" (June 18, 2014).

2. Center for Disease Control (CDC) statistics, cited in C. T. Arlotta, "How Obama Plans to Combat Prescription Opioid and Heroin Abuse in 2016," www.forbes.com, February 6, 2015.

3. Hazelden, 2014, "Parents in the Dark," http://www.hazelden.org/web/public/parents-drugs-children-survey.page (accessed October 21, 2014).

4. National Center on Addiction and Substance Abuse at Columbia University (CASA), June 29, 2011, "Adolescent Substance Use: America's #1 Public Health problem," http://www.casacolumbia.org/newsroom/press-releases/national-study-reveals-teen-substance-use-americas-1-public-health-problem.

5. CASA, June 2012, "Addiction Medicine: Closing the Gap Between Science and Practice," http://www.casacolumbia.org/addiction-research/reports/addiction-medicine.

6. Substance Abuse and Mental Health Services Administration (SAMHSA), "2013 National Survey on Drug Use and Health: Summary of National Findings," September 4, 2014, http://store.samhsa.gov/product/Substance-Use-and-Mental-Health-Estimates-from-the-2013-National-Survey-on-Drug-Use-and-Health-Overview-of-Findings/NSDUH14-0904.

7. Laxmaiah Manchikanti, "National Drug Control Policy and Prescription Drug Abuse: Facts and Fallacies," *Pain Physician*, 10 (May 2007): 403.

8. SAMHSA, "2013 National Survey on Drug Use and Health," 3.

9. NCADD, "Drinking and Substance Abuse Among Women in the U.S. on the Rise," http://ncadd.org/in-the-news/483-drinking-and-substance-abuse-among-women-on-the-rise (accessed 27 January 2015).

10. Rob Turrisi, Prevention Research Center at The Pennsylvania State University, *A Parent Handbook for Talking with College Students About Alcohol*, Tufts University, 2010, http://ase.tufts.edu/healthed/documents/parentHandbook.pdf.

11. National Institute of Mental Health (NIMH), *Women's Mental Health and Sex/Gender Differences Research*, June 20, 2003, http://grants.nih.gov/grants/guide/pa-files/PA-03-143.html.

12. SAMHSA/Center for Substance Abuse Treatment (CSAT), *Substance Abuse Treatment: Addressing the Specific Needs of Women. Treatment Improvement Protocol (TIP)*, Report 51 (Rockville, MD: SAMHSA, 2009): 17 and 74.

13. CASA, *Women Under the Influence* (Baltimore, MD: Johns Hopkins University Press, 2005), 45.

Chapter One

·········

My Daughter, Myself: Kim and I

"We parents see our children with a veil over our eyes," a top addiction research scientist shared with me over coffee. She wasn't talking as a scientist. She was speaking as the mother of an addicted child. And she was telling my story.

"Some experimentation is normal. Not all is pathological," the author of a well-known book about adolescent girls' growth in identity assures us.[1] (Not so reassuring is another passage where she describes how teenage girls are "going down in droves. They crash and burn in a social and developmental Bermuda Triangle."[2]) Of course it is every parent's wish that a daughter is just going through a phase, that she'll grow out of it —that, God forbid, it's not a drug problem. She's becoming a young adult, and the world is filled—as never before—with temptations. So, crayon-colored hair, piercings, tattoos, wild bursts of moods . . . I could live with that.

If only it were just that. One of the greatest tools a parent has in raising her child is intuition, but, as I and other parents share in this book, it can get lost in the tumult of dealing with teenaged angst. Time after time when talking to other parents of addicted daughters (many of whom are now in recovery), I've heard some variation of "I just knew something was wrong." But they didn't know what to do about it. That's what I told myself about my daughter Kim, at first as a whisper, later as a scream. Something was off, then way off, but what? Why? When I first noticed differences in Kim's interests, I felt that twinge. She'd loved playing the piano and she

1

had excelled as an ice skater. She was a diligent student with good grades. But at fourteen, these interests began to fade. At fifteen, she got kicked out of the all-girls school she had begged to go to, for taking stuff from other girls' rooms and hoarding it. No one was on hand when we went to pick her up on an icy February evening except a teacher's aide who suggested to me Kim was a kleptomaniac. And no one from the school ever contacted us after that to express any concern. We enrolled her in the local public school and got her into counseling. But Kim wouldn't communicate with us. She stayed in her room a lot. Her therapist explained to us she had self-esteem issues and that she had felt inferior to the many wealthy girls who were at her former school. This seemed an inadequate explanation to me, but she did appear to stabilize and made some new friends. So maybe the therapist was right.

When I found out a bit later she was smoking cigarettes, I was dumbfounded. Only two years before, Kim had begged her dad to quit smoking his nightly pipe, having learned of the dangers of nicotine in middle school. Of course we forbade her to smoke, but she just kept buying them from older kids and sneaking off to smoke. I now know it was the summer after her sophomore year in high school when Kim began smoking pot in earnest, drinking, and taking pills, as well as hallucinogens—"shrooms," or mushrooms—and Ecstasy, known as "Molly," while on overnight stays at friends' houses where, unbeknownst to me, the parents would cover for the kids. (In fact, she took all kinds of pills with her new buddies, sleeping pills they took from medicine cabinets or bought from other kids, such as Xanax, Ativan, what have you.) I didn't have a clue. I made a point of meeting Kim's new best friend's mom, a hardworking, friendly nurse with rosy cheeks. It was fine with the mom that Kim stayed over at her house frequently that summer. I had no idea she left the girls unsupervised or else drank with them. My husband and I found a bong in Kim's room and a half-empty bottle of vodka (we didn't yet know about the pills). So we grounded her. We had earnest, stern talks, we tried to encourage healthy interests. Kim was defiant, raging, sly, manipulative, always at least one step ahead of us.

Statistically, my daughter's experimenting with cigarettes, marijuana, booze, and other drugs as a mid-teen was on target. When puberty hits, besides depression, which can show up as a preoccupation with body image, girls (as well as boys) may have other issues manifest in adolescence, from bipolar disorder to ADD to other mental health problems. Kim was a late-bloomer physically and secretly agonized over her slow development. I didn't know how depressed she was. The therapist kept telling us she was working on her issues. And—I'm not proud of this—when I found out Kim was smoking pot and drinking, although I was upset, my attitude was mixed. Because I had done it, too. I remembered my own baby boomer youthful rebellion and angst, my own experimentation with loud music, hippie clothes, and drugs. I hoped I was helping her by telling her about my own use (a much-edited version), by emphasizing the problems drugs and alcohol had led to in my young life. Experts are divided about whether it's helpful to tell our children about our own history with substances. In Kim's case, what she heard from me was that I'd used different stuff and now I was fine. She simply blocked out all the trouble it had caused me.

My husband and I began to have conflicts over how to deal with Kim. She'll grow out of it, I assured him, she's seeing the therapist every week and we just have to be firm but not punitive. He was made of sterner stuff. He got angry at her antics, while I tried to understand. But neither of us really knew what to do. We cobbled out strategies, rules to lay down and stick by. But she was so defiant and such a good liar. In her junior year, I was relieved when she got a boyfriend. Tom seemed like a nice young man. He lived in a nearby town, with good parents and a kid sister and a horse. Tom was a guitarist and they were both huge movie fans, so it made sense to both sets of parents that they spent hours in Tom's family's finished basement with the flat-screen TV and stereo system. None of us knew what they were doing was spending hours stoned on Oxycontin, the powerful painkiller oxycodone hydrochloride.

I was still pretty clueless. Kim was never a "big" drinker, but she and Tom and their group got drunk occasionally. As I mentioned earlier, for young women, binge drinking, often coupled with eating disorders, is a serious, under-recognized problem that has increased in recent years. As for the pills, I had no idea kids in suburban, urban, and rural communities all around the country were finding prescription pain pills by the cartload in family medicine cabinets, or that they were sold illegally and easily available. At Kim's nice suburban high school, there was a thriving market in the parking lot. There probably still is.

We didn't know how quickly kids or anyone—there is a growing problem of addiction in older people, too, who are prescribed pain medication and become dependent on it—get addicted to opioids, especially Oxycontin, or "oxies." The abuse of oxycodone and other opioids like Percocet and Vicodin, which has frequently led to heroin addiction, killed more young people from overdoses than crack cocaine in the 1980s and heroin in the 1970s *combined*.

Kim was kicked out of Tom's house when his father discovered they were using oxies, and he was sent away to rehab, but we didn't know this for some time because we weren't told. Now she spent time with other artistic, bored, alienated kids, including older kids who'd already graduated, which I now consider to be a red flag. Sometime before her senior year, I now know, Kim began sniffing crushed painkillers and then heroin. Our sense that something was wrong was now chronic. She had endless excuses about where she was and what she was doing, which is what addicts do. When I discovered what she was doing I went numb with shock—I was shattered. In the '70s and '80s heroin use was looked upon with horror by baby boomers like me. It was and still is a strong taboo. Some of us didn't think twice about "experimenting" with pot and psychedelics when we were young, but the stigma attached to heroin was huge. It was for outlaws, gritty urbanites, and "minorities." Well, those days are over. A few years ago, drug companies were pressured, after many deaths from overdoses, to change the formulation of Oxycontin so it couldn't be tampered with to be crushed to snort or inject. Among women, deaths from prescription pill overdoses such as Oxycontin quintupled since 1999, to about eighteen women every day.[3] But once oxies were made tamper-proof, voilà, heroin became the alternative. In the immortal words of one high school student, "It's cheaper than a six-pack!" And this terrible epidemic has continued, an epidemic that so far mostly impacts young Caucasians, rich, middle-class, and working-class alike.

Let me tell you a bit about me. I'm an alcoholic who has been sober nearly forty years. I come from a loving, large family with a kind and hard-working father who hid his alcoholism for years, helped (endlessly) by my mother who was determined to keep that fact hidden, in order, as she explained to me years later, "to protect you children." (It didn't work, Mom, but I get it.) As a young teenager, I was ambitious in school, had a lot of friends, a boyfriend, and participated in lots of extracurricular and church activities, but underneath I felt more and more lonely, unsupported, and depressed—and increasingly "different." I drank along with the crowd in senior year at parties and dances, but it wasn't until I went away to college and discovered the "alternative" lifestyle of the '70s that I felt the thick fog of depression lift, some of the time at least. Because now there was cheap wine along with beer, marijuana, psychedelics, then a raft of drugs including cocaine, Dexedrine to study for finals, and other substances I've since forgotten. For a while, my new lifestyle of mostly pot and cocaine and drinking in bars made me feel smart, sexy, empowered. But addiction is a progressive disease. Although I was ambitious and loved to travel and had friends, within a few years I was isolated and drinking as much as I could, as often as I could, because I had to. Then the momentary easing of anxiety and heavy self-criticism didn't work anymore. I felt worse than ever. As many women addicts do, I rapidly became a blackout drinker. But I still didn't connect the trouble in my life with my using: the bewildering and complicated phenomenon of denial is a hallmark symptom of the disease.

The turning point came gradually for me. The final straw was a visit from my sister with whom I was very close. She told me lovingly, tearfully, but firmly just how my addiction was affecting her and my family. After a bit more of the paralyzing sense of aimlessness and fear I had gotten so used to and that continued to fuel my drinking, I hit a wall. I didn't want to quit using—but I didn't want to live the way I was anymore. This seemingly hopeless moment, when despair meets clarity, can be priceless for an addict, because it can lead to recovery. It was the late 1970s, and there were few options for treatment at that time. But my moment of clarity somehow brought me to the twelve-step meetings that turned out to be all over the place. I went to meetings with no idea of what I'd find, out of desperation. There I met people—especially women—who were calm and supportive and who told stories I could relate to. They gave me endless practical suggestions, which I desperately needed, on how to stay away from substances and learn to live a healthy life. Getting into recovery was painful and hard, but the healing has been worth everything. Along the way I met thousands of women and men with the same disorder who now have calm and productive lives. And these days more and more young people are crowding the rooms of twelve-step fellowships looking for a foundation for their life in recovery—as well as many other alternative support systems that didn't exist until recently.

You'd think, wouldn't you, I'd have recognized Kim's addiction sooner, given my history. I knew that, as one study puts it, "a genetic predisposition to addiction and/or co-occurring mental health problems [put kids] at greater risk of progressing from substance use to addiction."[4] Yes, I worried about that, but I also thought having a role model of a mother in recovery as an example of a disease that can be arrested with diligence would give her the necessary ammunition against the temptation to use when the time came. Wrong! Also, who could have predicted middle-class kids, with opportunities that most of the world can't imagine, would turn in such numbers to a drug that adults today associate with hard-core street users? And then there's that thick veil, that inability or unwillingness to see—the denial.

My daughter became bone-thin, either slept all the time when she was home, raged and cried hysterically, or disappeared. My husband and I stepped it up. We took away serious privileges. Then, in the spring of her senior year at an alternative program for gifted, alienated kids (most of them miserable and many on drugs), one of her teachers called me in for one of those "talks" I'd grown to expect and dread from the authority figures in her life. Usually, they talked about Kim cutting class, missing homework. But this teacher was different. She cut to the chase: Kim had a serious drug problem and we needed to get her help. Hearing the truth from another responsible adult—that Kim was actually "hooked"—was like having bandages ripped off my eyes. I had been distracted by the side issues, her slipping grades, her questionable new friends, her new, horrible temper, her arrests. I'd continued to see her as she had been, like looking at photos of the adorable little girl I'd doted on. "Miss Social Butterfly" in preschool. Lead in the school play twice. Brownies and Girl Scouts. Theater camp. Talented in a variety of artistic pursuits.

In my research I've read or been told time and time again that girls often escalate their drug use to deal with trauma. It can cover a range of experiences, from physical or sexual abuse to what they perceive as a life crisis. In our family's story, the escalation of Kim's drug use is tied to a major loss. After suffering increasing pain, her father was diagnosed with terminal cancer in the fall of her senior year in high school. By the time the teacher laid it on the line to me in the spring, he was in and out of the hospital and in constant pain. We knew he didn't have long to live and I determined to shield him from this painful news about his beloved daughter. I got her into an outpatient group for adolescents that met five nights a week at a local rehab center. At the weekly parents' meeting, where kids, moms and dads, and grandparents and counselors met in an enormous circle, Kim was soon speaking up articulately about how grateful she was to be giving up the drugs and finding healthy alternatives. Of course, I wanted to believe her so much. And she wanted to believe herself, I understand in retrospect. But she also tells me that before and after the outpatient sessions, there were kids selling drugs to each other in the parking lot.

With drugs available all over suburban New York she soon caved after her short "clean time" in outpatient treatment. Her addiction pulled her further and further away from everyone and everything she had liked. This is the bewildering beast at the heart of an addict's self-destruction. It is too painful and too frightening for the addict to think of stopping and it leads to bad decisions and terrible isolation.

Watching her vigorous, active, fun-loving dad crumble and eventually die a week before she managed to graduate from high school, Kim fell apart. When she stood before her class to give a presentation as part of the graduation ceremony, I watched the tears pour down her face and felt my own stream down on mine.

I was completely exhausted in body, mind, and spirit from caring for my dying husband, trying to deal with Kim, trying to be there for her grown brother, much less dealing with my own grief. That summer, I hardly noticed when she'd stay out all night and make up lame excuses when she got home. I simply reacted. When money went missing and I found sheets of paper on which she'd practiced imitating my signature to forge checks, I hid my checkbook, my wallet, my credit cards, and I changed the password to my bank accounts. I searched Kim's room obsessively for bits of tinfoil, doll-sized Ziploc bags, and syringes. Sometimes I would beg her to stop. Sometimes I just cried. So did she.

Did I make a lot of mistakes with Kim? Of course I did. But as I was to learn, I was doing my best with the energy and knowledge I had. A parent's basic instinct is to protect a child. What I didn't yet understand was I was not protecting her: I was protecting her addiction.

She was supposed to go to peer-support twelve-step meetings after the adolescent group ended, but I didn't know if she actually attended the meetings. I told myself she was and that this was a clear sign of her getting better. She'd been accepted by the college she wanted to go to and I thought this would be a positive move. She'd get away from all those sleazy friends and start a new, independent life. In October, when I visited her at her residence hall, though, there seemed to be no supervision of the freshman girls. The suite they shared was a mess. Soon after that, the dean of students called me to ask if Kim had dropped out since she hadn't been to any of her classes. I called and confronted her. That weekend, I drove her and her stuff back home. She'd have to get a job, I said.

Crisis management had become the new norm. And the worse things got, the more I hunkered down; fear became a constant poison in my heart, my brain, my joints. Kim did get a job, then she promptly lost it, got another, lost it. I kept on rescuing her, fixing up her messes—in short, I continued enabling her addiction. I remember one awful night when she swore she would stop using drugs if I would drive her to an ATM and withdraw four hundred dollars she had to pay a drug dealer who was threatening to harm her. So I drove her to the ATM machine. I felt impelled to protect her, and I wanted to believe she could straighten out with the right support from me.

Each recovery story follows its own arc. The path to long-term recovery is often not straightforward. Along the way, Kim went to therapy, two outpatient adolescent groups, an inpatient rehab, moved away, came back home, and then went to a second inpatient rehab and aftercare at a sober house. She then had several more relapses before she became serious about her own recovery. And that's not unusual for young people! (Nor for not so young people.)

Of course, I didn't know about the latest scientifically backed types of treatment that help women of all ages with addiction. I didn't know about the great deal of research in the last twenty years into the differences between female and male brains, hormonal functioning, and psychological needs; and that women are particularly vulnerable to trauma. I didn't know each individual facing recovery needs careful screening and the proper treatment. I was fortunate to stumble onto these discoveries when I was desperately searching for a new rehab. For some mysterious reason, I got into a conversation with someone I knew only slightly who worked at the bank I frequent. He had always seemed sympathetic and one day I ended up sitting in his office, spilling out my story. He in turn shared his addicted son's story with me, and how he happened to know about a small, women-oriented recovery center that his sister, a noted addiction researcher, had helped establish. (I have had too many of these conversations over the years to think they are coincidental. Many others have had them too. When we open up to possibilities, there is room for grace.) It was at that treatment center that Kim began the process of letting go of her fear and shame and trauma. She began to blossom. Though, as I say, she had relapses after that, Kim tells me the core experience of learning to trust herself and other women at the recovery center stayed with her. Getting into recovery is a process, and rehab is an important first step, but often it can be just that. Kim had to move far away from all the "people, places, and things" that tempted her in her home state, get a good sponsor—a woman with longer recovery who advises and supports a woman who is new to recovery through the inevitable growing pains—and open up to recovery because she wanted to. Her path has been full of the ups and downs of being a young adult, plus dealing with the aftershocks of active addiction, such as paying back her debts, dealing with health issues, emotional issues, and generally needing to acquire life skills. Today, our relationship is based on truths that were painful and hard-won for both of us. It was Kim who had to make the decision to get well. I had to learn to let her.

Accepting my child was addicted was the first of several difficult steps I had to take. Later came clarity about separating the addiction from the child and learning new ways to protect both of us from her addiction. That I couldn't fix her was one of the hardest truths I've ever come to terms with. But step by faltering step, it was also liberating. And it was essential in order for the healing to begin. How I wish I had known sooner how to love my addicted daughter more effectively. That is why I've written this book, to share a wealth of tools and tactics and information about treatment that best serves young women caught up in addiction. As parents and loved ones, let's arm ourselves with the most effective knowledge. And, just as importantly, let's avail ourselves of nurturing life-style changes. We can make the journey to peace of mind and offer the strong possibility of a healthy life to our kids. As one parent of an addict who is now in recovery, journalist Bill Moyers, said, "If your daughter came to you and said she had breast cancer, you would work out a way to have it treated. The same goes for addiction."[5]

It is us parents and caregivers who are on the frontlines when our children find themselves in trouble with substances. I hope this book will offer you hope as well as useful, practical support and guidance for both you and your daughter.

Notes on Chapter One

1. Mary Pipher, *Reviving Ophelia* (New York: Riverhead Books, 2003), 19.

2. Ibid.

3. Sabrina Tavernise, "Deaths in Painkiller Overdoses Rise Sharply Among Women," the *New York Times,* July 3, 2013.

4. National Center on Addiction and Substance Abuse at Columbia University (CASA), June 2012, "Addiction Medicine: Closing the Gap Between Science and Practice," http://www.casacolumbia.org/addiction-research/reports/addiction-medicine.

5. Bill Moyers, "Addiction Can Be a Disease and a Behavior," the *New York Times*, April 10, 1998. William Cope Moyers is the author, with Katherine Ketcham, of *Broken: My Story of Addiction and Redemption* (New York: Viking, 2006).

Chapter Two

. . . .

Does Your Daughter Have
an Addiction Problem?

"I think parents put on blinders," confides Amy. A young woman in her early twenties, she has been off drugs for a year and a half. She describes growing up in a loving home in a stable community. Then in high school, feelings of awkwardness about herself led her to try pot, and next the readily available prescription painkillers that were hawked around the school. By the time she graduated she was snorting heroin. Since Amy managed to keep up her work and got into college, her family thought she must be okay, if a bit depressed. It wasn't until she was arrested for possession of illegal drugs in college and faced significant jail time that they realized they had ignored a lot of troubling signs along the way.

Taking the First Steps toward Change

Will a parent see trouble ahead when they are reassured by signs of achievement, even if their daughter is withdrawn or moody or rebellious in other ways? How can we distinguish between a little experimenting, risky behavior, and abuse of alcohol or other drugs? Isn't it a rite of passage for kids to "experiment" a little? Isn't it usually just a phase? Many young people stick to "recreational" use at parties with their friends, and that's as far as it goes. Some parents who may themselves have indulged in their youth don't want to be hypocritical. They might even feel a bit nostalgic.

What you need to know: The possibility of a child's using drugs or alcohol usually begins around puberty. For girls, this age arrives increasingly earlier, and by age thirteen, "more than twice as many girls as boys are depressed, a proportion that persists into adulthood, regardless of race or ethnicity."[1] And depression increases the risk of addiction. It could be you become concerned about signs of depression in your daughter and seek help for her from a counselor or therapist. But a depressed young woman who is using substances is more likely to hide her substance use and to be treated for depression than for her drug use, whereas a depressed young man who uses substances is more likely to get treatment for his addiction. In fact, women of all ages are less likely to be diagnosed with addiction than are men.[2] Therefore, if your daughter is depressed, have her checked out by a competent physician for possible drug use. Many parents of young women using drugs I've talked to sent their kids to therapists. The girls were sometimes prescribed antidepressants—but their use of substances went undiagnosed.

There are, of course, many factors besides depression that drive girls to use substances. It seems parents have a different view of what motivates their children than the kids do. In one study, when asked to choose from a list of reasons why kids use drugs, most parents picked "peer pressure" or "it feels good." But their kids mostly chose "stress."[3]

Stress for girls and young women can coalesce around their body image. Lifestyle marketing bombards them with sexually charged ads that depict women as thin, thin, thin. Not long ago, the tobacco companies had tremendous power over young people's decision to smoke. Remember Virginia Slims? That power may have been curtailed, but it's going strong in the liquor industry. Ads infused with glamour show smiling (thin) young women sipping concoctions like the Skinnygirl Cocktail line. Or have you heard of alcopops, those cocktails on training wheels?

Illegal drugs, in turn, have won a subversive glamour of their own in America in waves of different epidemics over the centuries. I was surprised to learn the first big drug addiction epidemic occurred in the late 1800s, led by legally prescribed opiates such as laudanum, as well as patent or over-the-counter medicines that contained such additives as Coca-Cola syrup, which at that time included cocaine for a pick-you-up, marketed mostly to women to increase energy.

As Thomas Deitzler, Director of the Young Adult Program at the Caron Center for Recovery, put it to me in a conversation in 2010, "Addiction is in epidemic proportions with this generation." Again, the vast majority of risky users and addicts start when they are teenagers; women get addicted to alcohol and other drugs more quickly than men.[4] Yet they often hide their use more than young men do. "Boys learn from their earliest days on the playground, jumping at dares, that the willingness to take risks is part of what it means to be a man. For adolescent boys, alcohol and other drug use is the next step in the natural progression of risk taking . . . . Boys who drink may feel invincible, immortal, and beyond the reach of the law."[5] More often than girls, boys using substances may also seek negative attention, like being suspended or kicked out of school, getting arrested, driving too fast and having a car accident, until it becomes clear to those around him, sometimes including the criminal justice system, that he has a problem with substances.[6] Girls tend to be sneakier and more adept at hiding their use, at least at first. The sooner parents identify and respond to a problem-in-the-making with them, the greater the possibility these young women will have a chance to regain healthy lives.

Checklist of Warning Signs of a Possible Substance Use Problem

An eighteen-year-old high school senior, who was taking a variety of painkillers—whatever she could get from friends who mostly cadged them from family medicine cabinets or bought illegally obtained painkillers—describes herself then: "I grew thin and listless, stopped showering, and began sleeping at all hours." She adds that her parents didn't suspect drug use until she ended up in the emergency room after an overdose.

The following checklist can help you decide if your daughter may be either at risk for addiction or already addicted. No one can predict which kids will go down the road of addiction. Early intervention saves lives. For young people whose brains are still developing in the teen years and until about the age of twenty-five, some of these warning signs may seem to be the "normal" moodiness of a young person navigating the rocky passage to adulthood. However, if you recognize more than a few of them in your daughter there is cause for concern.

Physical signs

- Smoking (Does this surprise you? It did me. But, research consistently links smoking to depression—and depressed young people are more likely to turn to alcohol or other drugs.)
- Red, watery eyes, heavy use of eye drops
- Shaking hands, feet, or head, lack of coordination, clumsiness, stumbling, lack of balance
- Puffy face
- Paleness
- Vomiting
- Nausea
- Hacking cough
- Runny nose (not from a cold or allergies)
- Frequent nosebleeds
- Dilated pupils
- Alcohol on the breath, smoke on the breath, bad breath
- Rapid heartbeat
- Sores that don't heal
- Spots around the mouth
- Needle or track marks
- Excessive talking (motor mouth), hyperactivity, clenched teeth, slurred speech
- Marked increase or decrease in appetite, sudden loss or weight gain
- Burns or soot on fingers or lips
- Messy, careless appearance
- Avoidance of family dinners
- Sleep problems (too little or too much)
- Passing out, seizures

Behavioral signs

- Lower grades, skipping classes, lack of participation, loss of interest in extracurricular activities, hobbies, sports; complaints from teachers
- Many (or more) arguments with family or friends

- Emotional meltdowns: irrational and inexplicable mood swings—such as being friendly, then angry, sometimes violently so—ADHD, rebelliousness, inability to control impulses, paranoid thoughts, panic attacks
- Depression, anxiety, conduct disorders
- Stealing money; unexplained need for money; disappearance of valuables
- Lying, including asking others to cover for her
- Sudden use of air fresheners, incense
- Car accidents
- Marked withdrawal from family and friends
- Different friends—usually older; avoids introducing them to you
- Paraphernalia such as pipes, razor blades, vials, baggies, straws, rolling papers, rolled-up money, pill or alcohol bottles hidden in her room, purse, or car
- Overheard conversations that raise suspicions
- General lack of responsibility—failure to do schoolwork or chores, flimsy excuses for missed curfews or obligations
- Chronic defensiveness
- Trouble with the law for any reason
- Someone (siblings, neighbors, school officials) trying to tell you she is using drugs or drinking too much
- Thinking that drinking and/or using drugs isn't that harmful

Effective Conversations with Your Daughter Early On

If nothing on this list resonates for you, you may still be concerned about preventing a problem before it starts. Or maybe you still have that lingering gut instinct that something is off. There may have been an "incident" or two that doesn't sit right. Perhaps emotions have escalated between you and your daughter. No matter what the reason, parents can play a vital role in helping her make good decisions about using substances. Even if she's not using now, you can't assume

- she's not interested in drinking or drugging—the majority of high school students will try something before they graduate, and binge drinking and drug taking is rife on college campuses;

- she's already learned about it at school—with certain exceptions, schools aren't effectively teaching about today's reality;
- she won't listen to you—parents are known to be the number one source kids turn to for important information.[7]

As a starting point, when and how you talk to your daughter can make a big difference. You'll be more effective when you're prepared and focused on avoiding a confrontation. Kids are much more approachable when they are not tired, such as at the end of a school day or after a sporting event. Choose a time when you both are more receptive. It may be going together somewhere in the car, at a coffee shop, or at home if that's a comfortable place. Remember all kids are generally resistant to "the talk." You need to be caring, respectful and, as my daughter's kindergarten teacher used to say, "put on your listening ears." How you talk to her can mean the difference between her shutting down or opening up. Showing concern and respect for her are bouquets.

Many experienced counselors suggest opening up the conversation by asking about other kids she knows. If you begin with general concern instead of zeroing in on *her*, it will probably be easier for her to open up, or at least not shut down, than if she feels she's being scrutinized or judged. Is she worried about any of her friends? Ask her how so-and-so is doing. Let her know you understand some kids struggle with substance use, and that you are genuinely concerned for their welfare. If you do ask your daughter about her own use, you may not get a truthful answer, but you have set a tone and reminded her of your positive role. By doing so, you have opened up a new pathway that you can revisit.

Don't Dance with Her Denial

Let's say after one or more of these kinds of conversations with your child and a look at the checklist of warning signs you do suspect there may be more going on with her than the ups and downs of adolescence. Or that, again, you have that sense something else is wrong. Respect your parental intuition. But now what? It is a huge step to confront your child's risky substance use. Minimizing a suspected problem by making excuses for her drinking and/or drug use changes nothing, but a full-on confrontation usually does not work either. Demanding the truth from her can backfire. As one mother of an addicted daughter writes, "In my experience, denial, dishonesty, and manipulation are the behaviors most fundamental to addiction . . . . These behaviors become like second nature, helping the addiction take root and blossom."[8]

The operative word being denial—hers and yes, yours: an inability or refusal to face the truth because it is so painful and frightening, whether for the person who is addicted or her loved ones. The user becomes incapable of being truthful to herself about what she's doing. This is the aspect of addiction that may be the hardest to understand. When I was at the worst phase of my addiction, the need for the substance and the neurological distortions caused by the substance, degraded my ability to see reality to such an extent that using logic with me was pointless. My daughter, for her part, would explain away a slew of symptoms associated with addiction—irresponsibility in every area, extreme messiness, poor hygiene, high irritability, and deceitfulness—as being due to "teenage hormones" and "PMSing." (Ironically, she was partly right, as we do know sex hormones play a vital role in the emotional lives of young adult women.) Kim also played the moral outrage card: I was "invading her privacy." I was "a snoop." And my favorite: I was "bipolar." Like many other parents of addicted daughters I've met, she used lies and anger as weapons to fend off the truth. She lied because she was on the defensive and had to protect her addiction. For a while, it was effective.

When confronted about her use, a young woman is likely to minimize the problem or just lie about it. In scientific terms, the intake of booze or drugs increases the experience of pleasure and reward in the user's brain because more dopamine is being produced. Anyone who has a drink knows this feeling. But for the habitual user, there is a hazard: Over-stimulated by all those calls for dopamine, the brain of the heavy substance-user in time slows the process down by decreasing nerve cell proteins that function as dopamine receptors. It is then that the alcoholic or addict experiences a deficit of pleasure, tries to recapture that pleasurable sensation by drinking or using more in compensation. In short, a user needs more and more of the drug to recapture a sense of normalcy and, in short order, to avoid a mental crash since alcohol and other drugs drastically change the normal brain circuitry. In time, to feel just "okay" she has to get the next fix, which becomes a constantly diminishing okay, and in-between the lows get lower and lower. When backed into a corner, an addict guards her addiction as ferociously as a mama bear protects her cub. She'll view confrontation as an attack. This is the tough reality we have to face to be helpful.

Things kids who use drugs may say to protect their drug use:

"You don't understand."

"I'm just having a tough time right now."

"I've cut back."

"I can cut back."

"I will cut back."

"I can stop whenever I want."

"I'll deal with it when I find the right person/get the right job," etc.

But the truth may be quite different: She physically craves the pleasure—the "high"—and the escape the drug provides. Soon she needs the substance(s) she began using to feel more relaxed or to boost her energy or to forget her problems or just to avoid feeling terrible. Her brain-body chemistry now screams to avoid the physical pain of withdrawal.

During the initial period of my daughter's increasing use of drugs and alcohol I clung to the fiction that "things" weren't out of control. I kept hoping I'd overreacted and that with the right combination of discipline, activities, and friends, Kim would be alright. Following are comments from parents who, like me, got caught up in their own denial. Do you identify with any of the following?

"I wanted to believe her so much."

"Drinking with friends at that age was normal, as long as she wasn't driving drunk."[9]

"It was just marijuana."[10]

"It wasn't that bad."

"I allowed her to manipulate me."

"I covered up for her."

"I gave her money."

"I couldn't let her sit in jail."

"I should have set stricter limits."

"We let the problems in our marriage ruin our child's life."

"I kept trying to fix her problems."

"I sat at home worrying."

"The harder I tried to make her see the problem, the more she resisted."

"I was overwhelmed with everything because of what was going on in her life."

"I didn't talk to anyone about the problem."

"I didn't want anyone outside the family knowing about our problems."

"We kept giving her one more chance."

"I would know if my kid was using."

I said each of the above at one time or another. As parents, we want to protect ourselves from what is painful to accept in our children. As Kim's addiction worsened, I learned a vital lesson: By evading the evidence of my child's drug use, I was actually delaying the process of her getting well because there were no serious consequences to her actions.

We needed to have a different kind of conversation. We needed to communicate about consequences—positive as well as negative—for the choices she was going to have to make.

Samantha's Story

"Trauma," says Stephanie Covington, a leading expert on women and addiction, may be "any stressor that occurs in a sudden and forceful way and is experienced as overwhelming." She adds "Trauma also impacts how the brain functions. People under extreme stress often process and organize information differently." [11]

Pam and Neal have two daughters, ages eighteen and twenty-two, and live in a pleasant suburb of New York City. Pam, who recently retired because of a medical condition, worked as a Credentialed Alcohol and Substance Abuse Counselor (CASAC), both in outpatient and inpatient programs at a rehabilitation center. "I was shocked by the lovely young women getting into opiates," she says. "Many of them came from the courts. With the repeal of the Rockefeller drug laws, they could get treatment the first time instead of jail." These drug laws in New York State had been among the toughest in the nation. Repealed in 2009, they had required mandatory prison sentences for lower-level felons. "I remember one young girl especially. She had a very strict, loving family and she was a full-blown heroin addict by eighteen. The parents were overwhelmed. They couldn't believe it. And that was my story too."

Pam's older daughter Samantha was diagnosed with ADHD in the third grade. "She couldn't sit down or sleep. We tried everything else first before she finally went on Ritalin. It really helped: her behavior markedly changed. She still takes Ritalin. As a child, Samantha always wanted to get out and experience life. She had to be with the cool kids, she'd put up with them because status was so important. She's had big problems since she was a little girl, going to extremes sometimes. My younger daughter is not like that."

Pam and Neal started finding pot in her room when Samantha was around twelve or thirteen. "We'd find glass pipes, paraphernalia. The third time we found pot, she started going to a therapist once a week— someone I knew who worked at a recovery center. She was negative about it at first, but ended up enjoying speaking to her. And I didn't see more evidence of pot use. But then, at fifteen, she was arrested for shoplifting in Manhattan. She had to sit in a jail cell at a local precinct until we showed up. My husband wanted to hire an attorney so she'd get off, but I wanted her to face the judge and tell the truth. Well, she was given community service and had to work at a local library and at an arts program there on Saturdays, which was very good for her. She also went to an adolescent outpatient group program—where she was drug-tested—with a family group that met once a week. And she did well. After the group program, she continued to meet with a therapist one-on-one, then graduated to group peer counseling with a social worker and other adolescents—all of this for about eighteen months. In her senior year in high school, she went to an alternative program and got into the college she wanted at eighteen—a studio arts program.

"In college, she was in a dorm her first semester and did great. In the spring, she met a guy at a party who was about five years older than her and fell in love. First love. By the summer they decided he'd live with her in a student house at college. I always wanted to have an open relationship with her, so I was glad she was open with me about it. And he did keep her on point, academically. But as they started living together, I noticed

Samantha was becoming very thin. I was worried about her, and I asked if she was eating enough. Looking back, she was probably doing heroin then. The boyfriend was smart, but I knew he'd had a tough childhood. And then I found out he used to have a heroin problem, which he'd kicked. Well, that's what he said. It was probably BS. Meanwhile, he was buying her beautiful things: clothes, jewelry, and so on; I would see her modeling them on Facebook. And he didn't have a job. But she had been doing well in school, so . . .

"She stayed at the college after her sophomore year for summer school. But she wasn't answering my phone calls. When there was no bill from the college, I confronted her and she made some illogical excuse about why she wasn't going to school. In my gut, I knew something was wrong. Her dad was angry because she lied. We told her, 'You'll have to get a job for the summer if you are not going to school,' and she went and got one at a yogurt store. She would come home occasionally and she'd sleep in late, way into the afternoon. I didn't realize why: she was using heroin. My misconception about heroin was that you could not function because you would shoot up, go on the nod, then shoot up again, and continue the cycle. But, she was probably using it all the time just to be normal. I don't know if she shot up or snorted it because she still won't talk about that, but I found syringes in her room and in a car she and her boyfriend borrowed. They made excuses about it. I found three syringes in the spare bedroom from when Samantha, her boyfriend, and another friend visited. Again, there were the excuses. So I knew there was something wrong but I didn't know what it was.

"Samantha went back to her apartment at college in late August and one morning she calls me, absolutely hysterical: the police had come and taken her boyfriend away. He had become weird and paranoid—I later found out he had been doing all kinds of drugs. He started yelling at her, throwing stuff, and then he threw her against a wall and started choking her. Her roommate called the police. It was an automatic domestic violence charge. As the police were taking him away he assaults them. They took him to the ER, he was hospitalized, and then released to his mother.

"Now she's on the phone with me, out of her mind, so I stay on the phone with her and talk her down while Dad makes the three-hour drive to get her and bring her home. On the phone, she only raves about being assaulted. Nothing about the drugs. She keeps playing the part of the abused woman who needs help. We arrange for her to see a counselor and she gives the counselor permission to say only that 'Samantha's in over her head and needs support to open up to you.' We go with her to the next session and Samantha tells us: 'I've been using heroin and I need help.' She said later, 'If the assault hadn't happened, I would have gone on using.'

"I knew it was a medical condition. We got her to a psychiatrist who prescribed Suboxone and a medication for people who've been traumatized and she saw him every other day for a month. She wanted to live at home for a semester. We told her, 'You have to go to a twelve-step meeting every day; you have to do this for recovery.' She did go to a meeting where she met lots of kids in the program. But both Samantha and my husband told me I couldn't tell other family members about the addiction. And the therapist agreed. I questioned that—were we supposed to lie? I started going to twelve-step groups for help with the family situation. She went back to school in the winter and has continued with school since. She went to fewer and fewer twelve-step meetings. But she took on a new group of friends—smart young women.

"To her, it's like 'that part of my life is over now.' She's doing well in school, still taking the lowest dose of Suboxone and I'm still going to twelve-step meetings. It scares me that she doesn't deal with her addiction by continuing to participate in the fellowship. Samantha has lost two friends to drug overdoses. I'm in long-term recovery myself. From my twelve-step group, I've learned I don't always know what's best for Samantha. I need to keep the focus on myself. If I'm afraid or worried, it's not necessarily real. And I needed permission to help myself. I've learned I can be supportive from a distance and offer only suggestions. I will never go clean up her mess again—having to clean out her apartment after the assault at college and move her stuff made me physically sick. I became ill. The gift from that experience was realizing I couldn't do this for her anymore.

"I was the last child in the family to do the 'normal things.' I remember after entering recovery making amends to my mother (the Ninth Step of the twelve-step program). I told her 'I'm sorry I ruined your illusions of me.' And it's true: we write these scripts for our children. As for me, I don't want to miss seeing the addiction in my child if it happens again.

"For parents in a similar situation, here's what I've learned: Bring the child to a doctor for a check-up. Know the diagnostic criteria for substance dependence. If you feel there's something wrong, go to a good therapist or clergyman. If your child is arrested or has a DWI, get her help. Don't wait. You don't have to put up with unacceptable behavior. Find a support group. Joining my twelve-step fellowship was the best thing I did for myself."

Drugs Other than Alcohol That Are Swallowed, Smoked, Snorted, or Injected

Amphetamines: Biphetamine, Dexedrine, Adderall. (An amphetamine used to treat ADHD, Adderall was prescribed fourteen million times for those aged twenty to thirty-nine in 2011.[12])

Barbiturates: Amytal, Nembutal, Seconal, Phenobarbital.

Benzodiazepines: Among the most commonly prescribed Antidepressants, including Librium, Valium, Ativan, Xanax, Klonopin.

Codeine: Empirin with Codeine, Fiorinal with Codeine, Robitussin AC, Tylenol with Codeine.

Designer drugs: Currently cathinones (*bath salts*)—with effects similar to amphetamines and cocaine—and *cannabinoids* (K21/Spice), synthetic marijuana, are the most widely used in this class. Note this class of drug is constantly growing.

Dextromethorphan (DXM): An ingredient found in any cold medicine with "DM" or "TUSS" in the name. This one is over-the-counter.

Ecstasy or *Molly*: MDMA, a synthetic, psychoactive drug.

Fentanyl: A powerful opioid pain medication.

Flunitrazepam: Not approved for use by the Food and Drug Administration, which has not stopped its distribution in the United States, it is also known as Rohypnol. Commonly called "Roofies" or "Mexican Valium," it is the "date rape" drug.

Heroin: An opiate derived from opium, a naturally occurring substance. Highly addictive, it can be smoked, snorted, sniffed, or injected. Street heroin often contains toxic contaminants or additives that can cause permanent damage to vital organs.

Hydrocodone Bitartrate: Commonly known as Vicodin, although there are over 200 products that contain hydrocodone, including Lortab and Lorcet. This is the most prescribed drug in the country and the most abused.

Marijuana: Containing THC, it is the most common illicit drug in the United States. "A recent study of marijuana users who begin using in adolescence revealed substantially reduced connectivity among brain areas responsible for learning and memory."[13]

Oxymorphone: Opana, Numorphan, Numorphone.

Methadone: Methadose, Dolophine.

Methylphenidate: Ritalin, the most commonly prescribed central nervous stimulant used to treat Attention Deficit Disorder.

Roxanol, Duramorph: Morphine sulphate.

Other Opioid Pain Relievers: Oxycodone HCL: Tylox, Percodan, Percocet.

Hydromorphone: Dilaudid.

Phencyclidine: PCP, aka "angel dust."

Propoxyphene: Darvocet or Darvon.

Sleep Medications: Ambien, Sonata, Lunesta.

Tobacco: Cigarettes and other tobacco products contain the addictive drug nicotine and pose health risks. The additives to tobacco products are responsible for the most serious health consequences. The majority of young opiate users also use this harmful, if legal, substance. Recent research has shown it is harder for women to quit tobacco use than for men and that women benefit less from nicotine replacement therapy.

Zohydro ER: Long-lasting pure form of hydrocodone, and five to ten times more powerful than Vicodin.

Notes on Chapter Two

1. Anita Gurian, "Depression in Adolescence: Does Gender Matter?" Website of The Child Study Center, www.aboutourkids/org/articles/depression_in_adolescence_does_gender_matter (accessed January 27, 2015).

2. Susan R. B. Weiss, Hsiang-Ching Kung, and Jane L. Pearson, "Emerging Issues in Gender and Ethnic Differences in Substance Abuse and Treatment," *Current Women's Health Reports* 3 (2003): 245–53.

3. David Sheff, author of *Clean* (New York: Houghton Mifflin Harcourt, 2013) and *Beautiful Boy* (New York: Houghton Mifflin Harcourt, 2009), in his remarks at the sixth Drug Crisis community forum: "Hope and Recovery as We Confront Every Family's Nightmare—Prescription Drug and Heroin Addiction," hosted by Drug Crisis In Our Backyard and Phoenix House Academy of Westchester, Shrub Oak, New York, March 13, 2014.

4. National Center on Addiction and Substance Abuse at Columbia University (CASA), *Women Under the Influence* (Baltimore, MD: Johns Hopkins University Press, 2005), 46 and 74.

5. Dan Kindlon and Michael Thompson, *Raising Cain: Protecting the Emotional Life of Boys* (New York: Ballantine, 1999), 182–83.

6. Weiss, et al., "Emerging Issues in Gender and Ethnic Differences in Substance Abuse and Treatment," *Current Women's Health Reports*, vol. 3, no. 3 (June 2003): 245–53, http://www.ncbi.nlm.nih.gov/pubmed/12734036.

7. Rob Turrisi, Prevention Research Center at The Pennsylvania State University, *A Parent Handbook for Talking with College Students About Alcohol* (Tufts University, 2010), http://ase.tufts.edu/healthed/documents/parentHandbook.pdf.

8. Beverly Conyers, *Addict in the Family: Stories of Loss, Hope, and Recovery* (Center City, MN: Hazelden, 2003), 34.

9. Turrisi's research (*A Parent Handbook for Talking with College Students About Alcohol*) shows that teens who drink in high school drink more afterward.

10. Law enforcement officials report many tragedies of young people who smoke pot that was—unbeknownst to them—treated with other substances, such as PCP, or "angel dust." PCP was developed as an anesthetic but never approved for human use because of its intensely negative psychological effects.

11. Stephanie S. Covington, *Beyond Trauma: A Healing Journey for Women. A Workbook* (Center City, MN: Hazelden, 2003), 13. Reprinted with permission.

12. Alan Schwarz, "Drowned in a Stream of Prescriptions: Addict's Parents Couldn't Halt Flow of Attention Deficit Drug," *The New York Times*, February 2, 2013.

13. National Institute on Drug Abuse (NIDA), "Drug Facts: Marijuana," January 2014, http://www.drugabuse.gov/publications/drugfacts/marijuana.

Chapter Three

From Protecting Her Use to Helping Her Get Healthy

"I would tell parents and loved ones of a young woman showing signs of substance abuse that trying to talk reasonably with an addict about it will probably not yield the desired results. Love this person from afar. Treat her as if she had any other contagious ailment, because if you stay in close proximity to her you will absorb all her negativity and take on her problems as your own. She will try to manipulate you in every way possible. This is NORMAL! Your child has not become a monster; she has a disease. Help her reach her bottom faster by doing such things as cutting her off financially, making her friends aware of her condition, and changing the locks on your doors. These seem like dramatic measures. I assure you, they're not."

—My daughter Kim's advice to parents, after getting into recovery

Once I acknowledged, if not completely accepted (which took time and effort), my daughter's drug problem that she either denied or minimized, I knew I'd have to set limits and stick to them so as not to support the behaviors that were fueling her substance use. What kind of limit-setting has been shown to work?

If Your Child Is Exhibiting Risky Use
But You Don't Think She Is Addicted

The first thing I told Kim when I suspected she was using drugs—"just" marijuana, as I thought then—was that it was unacceptable. But experts who work with adolescents struggling with substance use say laying down the law like that not only doesn't usually work, it can even be harmful to your cause. Why? Your child may get sneakier and the deception piles on. Remember "Just say no?" That worked really well, didn't it?

In a culture that promotes having it all, where image is so highly prized, many young women don't know how to escape the peer pressure of "partying" even if they actually want to. Here are two "easy outs" we can offer that help them save face in a situation where their friends are urging them to use:

"I can't drink/use drugs because my parents do drug tests."

"I can't get high because I have a doctor's appointment tomorrow and they might take a urine sample."

Another strategy: Create a face-saving "code" she can use on the phone when she's stuck in an uncomfortable situation and wants to leave. For example, "But I'm not ready to come home yet." This kind of pre-planned arrangement serves two purposes: It tells you she wants to leave, and it won't invoke the ridicule or ostracism of her friends.

Setting Boundaries—Because Consequences Matter

A mother of a teenaged girl I know is accustomed to telling her daughter that curfew on weekends is midnight, even though she and her husband often stay out themselves until the wee hours. She can't understand why her child is rebellious. The father of another teenager likes to smoke pot occasionally outside, as he thought, discreetly. But he was furious when he found out his son was selling pot to other kids. I remember lying awake waiting for Kim to come home, then confronting her in her bedroom and threatening to take away the car keys. But I never did. Instead, I gave her another lecture and no follow-through. A few times my husband—who was more of a natural disciplinarian—found out and did take away her keys. Naturally, Kim played the divide-and-conquer game, deflecting our attention from her. He and I called a meeting with her therapist, who helped us realize we had to be a team and model consistency. And so, finally, we came up with a plan of what was and was not acceptable and what the consequences were.

After my husband passed away, I started seeing another counselor in the addiction field about Kim, who also helped me to cope with my grief. With his guidance, I went through another important learning process about my role in Kim's active addiction. I came to understand that while it is instinctual to want to defend and protect your child, when it comes to dealing with addiction we need to redefine our role. By letting her off the hook and shielding her from consequences your child will learn it doesn't matter if she breaks rules. This is one of the ways in which parents of addicted children can unwittingly love them to death. It is interesting to talk to kids in recovery about what rules mean to them. They may have fought rules tooth and nail, yet they consistently urge parents to enforce consequences and not cave in to their children because it's the easier, softer way.

Nobody should presume to know what are the right actions to take during the fraught time of a child's active addiction. For some parents, finding out their child uses alcohol or other drugs is so unacceptable they make the addict move out of the house. Others go bankrupt trying to deal with an addicted child. Still others ignore the elephant in the room, tiptoeing around it, unwilling or too afraid to admit or speak the truth.

I realized not only that I had to speak the truth and stick to my bottom line, but that I also needed to keep the conversation going with Kim for as long as it took, in a way that she could hear. I lost it with her sometimes. I would start out calmly and end up saying things like, "How can you be so inconsiderate, selfish, and irresponsible?" But I kept practicing my new way of talking to her. Gradually I learned to do the following:

- **Wait before speaking**—actually counting to ten—when she had done something to upset me. A calm tone gave me a sense of control and it gave her a chance to be less defensive and maybe even hear what I was saying.
- **Keep the focus on our boundaries**. For example, "I'm glad Isadora is coming over. Remember that at our house I stop by to talk to you guys every so often."

- **Be specific**. For example, "I could really use your help (with taking out the trash; emptying out the dishwasher, etc.)"
- **Be matter-of-fact**. For example, she'd say: "Mom! Dad! Don't you trust me?" And we'd reply: "It's not our job to trust you, we're your parents!"
- **Have clear rules.** For example, "No friends at the house when I am not at home."
- **Tell her calmly and specifically how her actions were affecting me and our family**. For example, "I feel so worried and concerned about your safety when you don't come home at night," "when you don't answer your cell phone" (and so on). "I am frightened something has happened to you."
- **Reinforce the positive in our lives, however small**. For example, "I'm so glad you have someone to talk to about your problems if you want to. When I was your age, I didn't have anyone," or "Your brother loved that dinner we had together the other night."
- **Stop forcing her to communicate in the moment**. For example, I'd say, "Let's talk this over when we both calm down."

I needed a lot of help to change the conversation—from a counselor, a support group, friends, and readings. I had to remind myself each day that the only way I could protect my daughter was by refusing to protect her addiction: By setting down clear consequences for her unacceptable behavior, but also never letting her forget I loved her. It hurt when Kim cried and raged at me when I took action if she failed to live up to her part of the bargain. I often felt like the worst mother in the world when Kim pleaded and begged for money. But I also kept encouraging her to do positive things. Kim has always loved to draw and keep a journal. I made sure to admire her artwork and talk about books we both liked, and I invited her to have dinner or go see a movie, even though she could sometimes be a no-show.

I knew I had to refuse to protect her addiction, but I reminded myself she was a frightened, lost young woman who badly needed encouragement and fun in her life.

Removing Temptation from the Home

Sometimes we fail at basic common sense. Kim's father was very ill for about a year before he died and needed to take ever-stronger pain medication that I hid in the back of a hall closet where I thought it would be safe. There came a heartbreaking day when he really needed a strong painkiller prescribed for cancer patients, but I discovered it was gone. I'd hidden it but didn't lock it up, and so of course, Kim had found it. Many studies have shown young people use alcohol or other drugs easily available in the family medicine and liquor cabinets, including that of grandparents and other relatives or from friends' parents' cabinets. Others become addicted after being given prescribed painkillers following dental work or a sports injury.

After surgery to reset a broken wrist, I was given a prescription of Vicodin. I had informed the surgeon I was an alcoholic in recovery and didn't like to take mood-altering chemicals. The doctor smiled and replied, "Trust me, you will need some Vicodin when you wake up from surgery." He was right, I did need strong pain relief for a day or two—but a whole bottle? No. I crushed the remaining pills in a paper bag and put them at the bottom of the garbage can, covered up with coffee grounds and other trash. The doctor hadn't told me how to dispose of the pills; a friend who works with addicts did.

Modeling a Healthy, Honest Lifestyle

Drinking or using drugs to blunt the pain of my family situation wasn't an option for me, but I did have a prescription bottle of sleeping pills for when I really needed them, and of course, Kim found those. That was another lesson. As for alcohol in the house, if you are concerned your occasional cocktail or nightly glass of wine might impact your daughter's recovery, choose to keep a dry household while your child is struggling with substance use or abuse: alcohol is a trigger, even if not the drug of choice. Some of us discover when dealing with a loved one's addiction that we are self-medicating too, and that it might be a problem. "Seeing a parent drunk raises the odds the child will drink excessively," concludes a survey of 5,700 schoolchildren in Great Britain, and there are plenty of other surveys that concur.[1] Your heavy drinking as a parent can lead to a greater risk of addiction in your children. Remember also the 40 to 50 percent increase in the likelihood of a child becoming a substance user if the genetic component for addiction runs in the family, as it does in mine.

Offering an example of sobriety, vitality, and integrity is a tremendous gift for a child in crisis. Getting support from and connection with other people in the same situation can be a great source of strength. Families similar to your own are out there in droves, and they are people who are motivated to maintain a positive outlook and peace of mind despite their child's addiction. I happen to be, well, stubborn is the word I'll use, but eventually I did cave in to the suggestion I'd been receiving from many people who cared about me: Go to Al-Anon! (Al-Anon is the fellowship for relatives and friends of alcoholics; Nar-Anon is its equivalent for addicts). I thought, "What, another twelve-step group in my life? These people are just going to depress me even more." Hearing more about the woes of addiction in families seemed like the last thing that would help me. But drag myself to a meeting I did. Surprise: I had a hard time accepting there that I too was sick from Kim's addiction. That it truly affects everyone within shouting range of the addict. Initially I thought, *Look, I have gotten well from this disease of addiction, and this is* her *problem. I'm willing to help her but* I *am okay. Kind of . . . well, maybe not.* So I kept going to those meetings, where it soon registered that everyone in our family was affected by Kim's addiction. And that all of "those" people in the fellowship were going through similar things. I was suddenly meeting people in the same situation as I was who were focused on getting healthy, on regaining some kind of peace of mind instead of obsessing about how to overpower their child's or their spouse's addiction. I received wise, practical suggestions about *my* needs and wants. Soon I found people I knew socially, from church, from a book club, from the gym, or from chatting with a neighbor at the grocery store, who had a family member with a problem with addiction—and, sometimes, there was a happy ending. My shame was lifting. It turned out there were endless sources of support for me once I became willing to open up. Some of these folks had a hard-won calm acceptance, a loving detachment they'd learned to apply to their relationships with addicted loved ones—whether they got well or stayed sick. And I wanted that; I burned for it.

My new twelve-step fellowship taught these essential truths:
- I didn't cause my daughter's problem, and it's not my fault.
- Her problem didn't happen overnight, and it's not going to be resolved overnight. (See the Appendix for the many free support groups for parents and families of an addict.)
- Other children in the family are a special concern. To one degree or another they become collateral damage. They are witnesses, they are frightened or angry or become withdrawn. Sometimes they are forgotten about in all the turmoil. My grown son and other close relatives lived halfway across the country, but on visits, Kim's self-destructive behavior hurt and bewildered them. I shared what I'd learned with them. Some accepted it; others did not, as is their choice.

For younger children, counseling or twelve-step groups specifically for teen family members of addicts can help them learn to express their own feelings, often guilt and anger, and develop healthy attitudes. Learning about the disease of addiction is a great benefit to them, both to understand their sibling and for themselves. As one expert who works with kids warns us, "Research shows that the risk for alcohol and other drug use skyrockets when children enter the sixth grade, between the ages of twelve and thirteen. To be effective in preventing alcohol use by teenagers, we must reach out to and educate children in grades one through five."[2]

After I had been to some twelve-step meetings, I began to want my life back. I had stopped doing many enjoyable activities and had become isolated. Also, like everybody else, I had lots of responsibilities apart from Kim. I had neglected family, friends, my work, the house, the garden I loved to get dirty in, even my beloved dog. I did simple things, like having lunch with a friend, joining the YMCA, weeding a patch of garden—even cleaning the pantry became therapeutic. I was still filled with shame and guilt and worry, but by entrusting a few people with my concerns and looking outside my narrow predicament, space opened up just for me.

Not everybody in my community and family was supportive. While the stigma against women substance users has lessened somewhat over the past decades, it's still strong. Certain friends backed away when they learned of Kim's addiction. Maybe they felt threatened or didn't want to be around me when I was not at my best. So I focused on the ones who were there just to have a cup of coffee with me, to be my friend and my little sturdy support network.

Coming to terms with my daughter's addiction and my role in it also gave me the energy to renew my spiritual discipline. Spirituality can be anything from sitting on a rock looking out on a forest to practicing a formal religion. Prayer and meditation reinforced a deep truth for me: Worry doesn't prevent disaster, it prevents joy.

Keeping the Communication Going

Kim and I had been in limbo, suspended in pain and conflict, for several years. As my thinking about her addiction changed and I felt better, I paradoxically stopped pretending everything was going to be okay—especially if *I* didn't rock the boat. I still hated the anger she vented when I gave her consequences, and I hated the anger that welled up inside me. Sometimes I still argued or pleaded with her. But it was no longer a blame or shame game. Kim's illness wasn't my fault, and I wasn't a failing parent. She was a very sick girl, and she did stupid, sometimes illegal things because of it.

When I hear our addicted children being called "bad kids" or "throwaways"—once even "garbage"—and that it's their "fault" they are addicts, I think of Peter. He was a pimply faced young man of eighteen in Kim's adolescent outpatient therapy group, a heroin addict. His parents had thrown him out and Peter lived by scavenging and stealing to feed his addiction. He broke down crying on my couch one night after I'd invited him to the house for dinner. A month or so later, he was caught stealing and went to jail for several years. And I think of Kim's friend Heidi, a defiant alcoholic and pill-popper, whose mother alternately spoiled her and screamed verbal abuse at her when she herself—the mother—was drunk. Her dad stuck his head in the sand, working long hours to escape the situation. As of this writing Heidi has lost her way and does porn for drug money, but I pray she can find the recovery she so desperately needs.

The medical and therapeutic community knows addiction is a disease: advances in studying the brain have made that clear. But society in general still stigmatizes addiction, and it is easy for a parent to do the same.

Young addicts, some not even old enough to vote, need to learn to love themselves and be responsible, not be punished for making bad and potentially fatal choices. And it's critical to involve the family in healing these young people. Kids like Peter and Heidi, unsupported or abused by their families, have a much lower chance at getting well. Many addicts expect to be judged and scorned, to not be met with compassion. They expect to hear, "What's wrong with you?" and not "What's troubling you?" I remember how concern and loving honesty—not lectures and guilt-trips—created a safe space within me where I could begin to hear the saving truth about my own addiction. Addicted children pile more than enough shame and blame on themselves.

As I practiced being matter-of-fact and nonjudgmental, firm but loving, with my daughter, I found I felt more adult—more in control of myself as a parent and as a person. And since I was no longer combative with Kim but simply stating the feelings her behavior aroused in me, she couldn't deny them.

That made her wary—she was still an addict, after all—and I was counseled I would need to keep having these new conversations for as long as it took. When I slipped into old nagging and pleading, all I had to do was acknowledge it and resume the new way of communicating. For instance, one day when she was still using, Kim found my hidden car keys and took the car while I was asleep. The next morning, I found my car with two shredded tires. Adrenalin poured through me. Forgetting about deep breaths, detaching, and being adult I stormed into her room and shook her awake. "How could you?" I shouted, slamming the door.

It's appropriate to get angry in situations like this. Yet I didn't want the old pattern of yelling at Kim to be the only consequence of her careless, thoughtless actions. So I went back in her room and told her in a firm, calm manner I would not make the mistake of forgetting to lock up my car keys again because she was not a responsible driver. If she wanted to drive, she'd have to come up with the money for two new tires. There was a direct and logical consequence of her behavior.

Offering Choices

Instead of giving orders or making demands, I was offering her a choice: the option of changing her behavior to get a reward. This empowered both of us. They were small steps, sure, but the dynamic between us improved. Want to drive the car? Pay for two new tires. Want to live in a pigsty? Fine, I am no longer your daily maid. I'll just keep the door closed.

By changing the dialogue, I gave Kim the opportunity to become responsible for her actions—not just negative consequences. "You catch more flies with honey than with vinegar," and addiction is all about negativity: from losing your friends, your self-esteem, to not even being able to get high anymore. It's important to provide addicts with logical rewards and encouragement when appropriate. (For more on this, see the CRAFT Program, as one example.[3]) Always let your troubled child know she is loved, because underneath the drugs and the defiance and the sullen withdrawals she has few if any positive feelings about herself.

Have an Overdose Plan

An eminent group of addiction therapists advise family members of anyone who uses opiates/opioids (Percocet, Vicodin, fentanyl, Oxycontin, or heroin) to be prepared in the event of an overdose. This includes those who use "recreationally without dependence."

The signs of opiate/opioid overdose are: blue lips and/or fingertips, loss of consciousness, strange snoring or gurgling sounds, slow breathing (less than eight breaths per minute) or no breathing.

What to do: Learn rescue breathing. Laws about making naloxone rescue kits (including nasal inhalers) are evolving quickly, so talk to your doctor about obtaining one. They are simple to use.

We always want to discourage her substance use and encourage her to make healthy choices, yet we want to be able to save her life if need be. We must hold her accountable, but blaming the addict usually only helps the addiction proceed. Anger and shaming might relieve our feelings for the moment, but a new kind of loving her—tougher, but respectful love—gives her the chance to change. The goal is always recovery of her health and well-being.

Terry's Story

It's estimated about 1.5 million of our twelve- to seventeen-year-olds meet the criteria for admission to alcoholism treatment, and 1.4 million for drug treatment.[4]

Elizabeth is a landscape gardener and fitness enthusiast who lives in a semi-rural suburb of a big city with her second husband Ben. She has identical twin girls, Terry and Penny, twenty-one years old. Elizabeth and their father divorced when the twins were seven, and they have lived with Elizabeth since. They see their father, who moved several hours away, infrequently. When the twins were eight, Elizabeth began dating a friend from high school, who became her second husband soon after.

"Terry has had a lot of anger toward her father, which she manifested once she got into high school. The girls grew up in a small town. At fourteen, when she was a freshman, Terry took the train to a nearby city with her close girlfriend on weekends to hang out at the mall. I've always encouraged my girls to be independent and it was okay for her to take the train. She had the option of coming home by 9:00 p.m. and we'd pick her up, or else she would have to walk home, which was not that far. But she'd be home by 9:00 p.m. She made friends with a group of kids at the mall, an Emo crowd, like Goth light—the black clothes and makeup, but not as extreme. Kind of dubious kids. But her friends were always welcome at our house.

"All that winter of her freshman year Terry went to the mall. And she started having panic or anxiety attacks. She smoked cigarettes and covered it with perfume. I didn't know. But I began to feel something was awry. She was hyper, always wanted to leave when we'd go places, like to an aunt or uncle's house; she'd want to get home. I didn't know she was high and couldn't sleep and had anxiety. She'd want me to come sleep in her bed. Then I found some pills in her room, and I suspected they were diet pills. I was just sick. I took them to the police and they said, yeah, they probably are. I found pills again, a prescription bottle—not hers. I called the pharmacy and they reluctantly told me that yes, they were diet pills. Terry never had any money, even though she got a good allowance from her dad. Yet she was still functioning, going to school, and then to dance classes afterward, but there was free time in there when she was probably hanging out with the Emo kids. Later I found out about these parties where the kids would have big bowls of all kinds of pills and just take them. And somewhere in there—Terry and I don't talk about it—I think she was date-raped. Something bad happened.

"There was a terrible night when Terry was at a sleepover, and her sister Penny was in a car accident. Terry came home in the morning wasted. It was horrible. And Penny's in the hospital and I had to get Terry packed for this trip to Europe for a program called People to People. Well, she was fine while she was in Europe, but when she came back she got involved again in the drug world. This time it was pot and cocaine—so dangerous when you're not quite fifteen. One morning during Labor Day weekend, she had a terrible anxiety attack with palpitations and she could hardly breathe. I had to take her to the ER. They stabilized her, but told me nothing about whether she was on drugs. Terry hid it. But the ER was a turning point for us. Things came to a head. I suggested she see a therapist and she agreed. She went to a psychologist. The psychologist told me she asked Terry what was going on, and Terry told her, 'There's certain things I want to do Mom objects to.' The psychologist said to me, 'Sometimes moms have trouble letting kids have the freedom they want.' But after the session, the psychologist recommended Terry see a psychiatrist.

"It's really hard to find a good one and they are expensive. Fortunately, her dad was able to pay. The psychiatrist created trust with her and left me out of the equation. For example, when I found a little bag of coke I stormed into his office and he told me, 'You can't put her under siege like this.' But he and Terry and I agreed I could drug test her, which I only did once. Terry turned out to have undiagnosed ADD and now she was being treated for that. Her meds were fiddled with, and sometimes she still felt panicky and needed to go off by herself and have a cigarette. But at fifteen, she quit using. The psychiatrist said there is a difference between risky use and abuse, and it was very helpful for me to hear that.

"Then we found out Terry was cutting—and this was after she had quit using. She had hurt her leg and needed to see a doctor. The orthopedic surgeon saw the cuts she'd made and said she couldn't release Terry to us unless the psychiatrist said it was okay, which he did. Otherwise, she would have been admitted to a psychiatric facility.

"Her twin, Penny, was a great help. She was able to explain to me what had been going on. It was a huge burden for Penny and it made her anxious. She had to take care of her sister, but she felt shut out too. Penny had told her dad before she told me, but he didn't do anything about it. He and Terry had a huge fight. There was much unpleasantness and pain. Penny watched the whole thing. So we got Penny into therapy also.

"Their stepfather was a rock. He's somewhat hands off with the girls but gives them unconditional love. He saw more of what was happening, he knew more, but he wasn't altogether sure of what was going on either. He didn't discipline the girls, I did. And he wasn't their confidant. His role was more as my support. And he was so worried about me. My stomach would churn and my heart was in my mouth. I was in a state of panic, too.

"Both of the girls are still working through things, such as their relationship with their father. They both have body image issues. As far as their education, Terry did okay in high school, but she has excelled in college. Penny always did well in school. They're both near the top of their classes. Terry has been accepted into a top school to pursue her master's degree. She remains drug free, and continues to see her psychiatrist as needed, who monitors her medication for ADD.

"She still has anger issues regarding her father and gets stressed out fairly easily, but is emotionally healthy and ready for adulthood. She wants to be involved in assisting female victims of abuse.

"Her sister, Penny, has begun her master's at an excellent school too. She continues to see her psychiatrist and plans to begin talk therapy soon to sort out her romantic relationship needs. She had an abusive boyfriend and wants to explore why she was in that relationship for so long. Penny is emotionally stable and is making her contribution to society as well.

"What I wish is that I had listened to my gut and done something sooner. I had my blinders on. I felt guilty and stupid. If a parent suspects drug use, get the child to a professional right away. I don't know how useful it is to talk to schools, I think a lot of them stigmatize kids. Get help and talk to someone—both for her and yourself. I wish I'd had someone to talk to. The signs were all over the place but I didn't see. When we did realize there was a problem, we got the ball rolling."

Notes on Chapter Three

1. Jenny Hope, "Children Who See Parents Drink 'More Likely to Binge,'" *Daily Mail*, June 17, 2011.

2. Mothers Against Drunk Driving (MADD), "Protecting You—Protecting Me," an alcohol prevention curriculum for schools developed by MADD (www.madd.org). For more information see: http://www.nrepp.samhsa.gov/ViewIntervention.aspx?id=95.

3. See also Jeffrey Foote, et al., *Beyond Addiction: How Science and Kindness Help People Change* (New York: Scribner, 2014).

4. Hazelden Recovery Center, October 5, 2011, "Hazelden expands outreach, services to help America's youth find recovery from drugs and alcohol" (Press Release), http://www.hazelden.org/web/public/pr111006.page.

Chapter Four

· · · · · · · ·

Providing Her with
Opportunities to Change

Drug Tests

Are drug tests an effective deterrent? Is it an accurate read of a child's suspected problem with substance use? Drug testing is one of the first things worried parents turn to when they think their child might be using. They buy a urinalysis kit (there are pages of them listed for sale on Amazon) and have their child use it in the bathroom. Sometimes it confirms their suspicions. But there are practical problems with this approach: A drug test won't show how often a child is using or how much, and many kits can't screen for certain illicit drugs that clear the system pretty quickly and won't be picked up on a general test. It's also fairly easy to "cheat" on urine screenings. Kids' creativity in thwarting tests is impressive. One example I read about involved the worried parents of a teenaged daughter who was caught "experimenting" with a variety of substances (cough medicine, Ecstasy, pot, and cocaine). They wanted to respect her privacy so they allowed her to close the bathroom door each time she had to urinate into a drug test cup. She would squeeze bleach into the cup from an eyedropper she'd hidden in the room, thus stymieing the detection of drugs every time.[1] A second example I know about from Kim, who learned of it during her stint at an outpatient program where she heard boys boasting about hiding fake penis tips with a tiny bag of "clean" urine—devices they'd bought online and hid on their bodies.

Putting the problem in the hands of a doctor—and preferably an addiction medicine specialist—means she'll get more sophisticated testing in a controlled environment and thus a more accurate outcome on the drug test. It also means you won't have to be the primary "enforcer"—not only a thankless task for any mother or father, but one that can damage the parent-child bond. "You are a parent," my therapist pointed out to me when I was struggling with this issue, "not a cop." I was advised to emphasize to Kim that testing for drugs is a safety issue, not a trust issue. Yet it's hardly surprising when a young person asked to take a drug test resists. Once she's eighteen, she can legally refuse to be tested. So be prepared with consequences. The calmer you can be during these conversations, the more likely it is she'll hear you. You may decide to revoke her driving privileges, not pay for schooling, and so on. Whatever you do, revisit the issue of drug testing if you think it's important.

Assessment by the Right Professional

The importance of who does the test cannot be overemphasized. It is natural to turn to the family doctor for advice on how to treat suspected use of drugs or alcohol. But many of these doctors have little if any training in recognizing or treating addiction—only 6 percent of pediatricians, for instance—although the American Academy of Pediatrics issued a policy statement in 2011 that doctors should routinely screen their teenage patients for drug and alcohol use at every visit, and look for signs of dependence or addiction. According to one addiction medicine specialist, "Despite the availability of [new] evidence-based prevention and treatment strategies, only a small fraction of individuals receive prevention or treatment consistent with scientific knowledge about what works."[2] Addiction medicine specialists and addiction psychiatrists receive additional training to identify substance use/addiction and to recognize and treat psychological or physical complications of the disease. As of 2011, there were 2,555 physicians listed as certified in addiction medicine nationwide, and roughly

2,000 psychiatrists certified in addiction psychiatry. Listings of these doctors by state are provided on the websites of the American Board of Addiction Medicine (ABAM.net) and the American Academy of Addiction Psychiatry (AAAP.org).

In a culture that places tremendous importance on self-reliance it is still healthy and essential to turn to others, to a community, especially when we have a crisis.

Thinking About (and Rethinking) Intervention

Senator George McGovern explains from his own experience with an alcoholic daughter that intervention is one way to bring about a "bottom" before something tragic happens.[3]

Yet some of us may be loath to act. We may think our options are limited to forcing her to go to some kind of treatment plan or else stage a full-scale intervention. We may not be clear about what intervention is designed to accomplish. Isn't it an invasion by a stranger (albeit a trained stranger) of the loved one's privacy—and also the family's? Isn't it a way of ganging up on her, attacking her when she's down? Hasn't everyone in the family gone through enough shame without some outsider's judgment?

CRAFT: Community Reinforcement and Family Training

This well-regarded evidence-based program teaches family members the use of healthy rewards to encourage positive behavior in an addict and to reduce or end substance use as well as to develop skills to take care of themselves. The program aims to help parents reduce relationship conflict through making small but important positive changes. CRAFT warns if the loved one is using drugs rather than alcohol, parents should reach out to a therapist or doctor as well, since the dangers of drug use can escalate more quickly.[4] The difference between reacting negatively to an addict by meting out punishments on the one hand and supporting her efforts to do positive things in her life on the other, can get fuzzy. One person's encouragement can be another's enabling. What helped me on a practical level was sound advice and support from people who understood this difficult, often overwhelming challenge for a parent. I needed support to be reminded that I was offering her love and respect by refusing to enable her addiction any longer, and that I was giving her the tremendous gift of hope for recovery by offering her ways to get well.

I like to call this *loving her back to life*.

Asking a Loved One to Get Treatment

You may decide you want to act immediately—to intervene. There are many ways to do so. Intervening can be as simple (though rarely as easy) as requiring your child to seek screening and then counseling. This counseling could be in the form of "brief interactive sessions directed at changing a substance-using adolescent's behavior . . . [ranging] from simple advice for low-risk adolescents to brief or short-term counseling for those at higher risk."[5]

If your daughter is a college student who is willing, look for a recommended prevention program. One such program, Brief Alcohol Screening and Intervention for College Students (BASICS), has had good results in curbing potentially dangerous practices such as binge drinking. Nonconfrontational, it consists of two one-hour interviews between the student and a professional. The program has been adapted for use with heavy marijuana users and with high school students as well.

There are other kinds of intervention that, when planned and conducted properly, can help a young woman who is at risk or substance-dependent. Sometimes more than one such intervention may be necessary. This was the case with Kim. She eagerly agreed to attend an alternative high school program off campus designed for at-risk college-bound seniors. (Some communities offer programs that address the varied needs of troubled teens within the school district. It's the same curriculum but taught differently. School guidance counselors should know about these opportunities.) While the program was beneficial, it wasn't enough. It helped her graduate and gave her needed skills and emotional support—but her drug use continued. She also attended that group outpatient program for teenagers at a local rehabilitation center, as well as individual counseling. But she continued to go back to using drugs.

Crisis-driven Intervention

Sometimes life itself intervenes with a crisis, such as an addicted child's getting arrested or suffering a medical or emotional emergency. Maybe it's the first time something like this has happened to her, or maybe it's just the latest in a string of emergencies, the one you decide is one too many. Young people—particularly young men, but women, too—will often end up involved with the criminal justice system. The good news is more and more judges and prosecutors today want to help stop the using in order to stop the criminal behavior. This may include mandated treatment in lieu of or before sentencing.

Because these crises can blindside parents, it is wise to do some advance homework about what facilities are available in your community and at large. Chapter Five will provide you with information to help make an informed decision about the type of treatment and facility you and your family may choose.

I personally hit the crisis button when I found drug paraphernalia, yet again, in my daughter's car after she'd completed her outpatient treatment—yes, you are entitled to snoop: This is about her life. At that point it seemed to me she didn't stand a chance as long as she stayed in her familiar surroundings where all her old drug contacts were in place. Our middle-class suburb swarmed (and continues to swarm) with the three things young addicts need: cash, drugs, and drug-taking peers.

My crisis intervention boiled down to a short talk—we had been on this merry-go-round so many times already. I had some examples, from other parents, of what to say, such as:

"If you go to treatment and show you're working at it, you can have your privileges back. What do you want to do?"

Or:

"If you don't go to treatment, you will have to make alternative living arrangements."

I expected to meet with resistance again. But it just so happened the timing was right; my daughter was ready to start facing her demons. The next day she was on a plane for an extended stay in (her second) recovery center. I wish I could tell you that that was the end of it, but it was not.

Young people tend to struggle with the chronic illness of addiction, and she was no different. However, it was a great new beginning for us.

Professional Intervention

You may decide you need the help of a professional interventionist in prying your daughter away from her addiction. Some background on this: In the early 1960s, Vernon Johnson, a recovering alcoholic and Episcopal priest, challenged the idea that a substance user has to hit "rock bottom" before she or he can be helped. His idea of interrupting the downward spiral of addiction led to the formation of a new profession called "interventionists." The Johnson Institute has since trained thousands of interventionists (it transferred its key components to the Hazelden Recovery Center in 2009). The process works like this: Family members and other loved ones meet beforehand, usually for five family sessions, with the interventionist. Together they decide

- the form of the intervention;
- who is to be involved;
- education and treatment plans; and
- the intervention plan.

The interventionist and family, perhaps with close family friends or affected others, then surprise the substance abusing family member with a meeting to discuss the effect of the abuse on everyone, the love and concern the family has for her, and the choice of treatment they propose. The family member who is using substances does not know anything about the intervention beforehand.

Two other types of professional intervention focus more heavily on the whole family. One, known as Family System, or Family Model Intervention, aims to help family members regain their equilibrium and health—even if the addict in the family refuses to change. It helps families understand and address how they have been drawn into a pattern of dysfunction. Often, one parent takes on the role of protector, also known as chief enabler, while the other parent (or family member) may be the enforcer, expressing anger and frustration about the child's addiction. Sometimes partners switch roles. The Family System Intervention works toward creating a united front in addressing the crisis with the child. The second type is Invitational Intervention, also known as ARISE. It too emphasizes family involvement, but is different in that it does not "surprise" the addicted family member; rather, it "invites" her to be part of the process. Evidence about which type of intervention is most effective is largely anecdotal.

A professional interventionist is not there to pass judgment on anyone, but to help the family get focused and resolved. All kinds of strong feelings can arise during the intervention process. The goal is to help a family stand firm despite the objections and manipulations of the addicted loved one. The interventionist guides the family to understand that the situation in which the active addiction has thrived must be removed. A typical example is providing material aid with which the addict is free to continue to find and use substances. The parent enabler (like myself) must be willing to cut off aid to the addict except for treatment. This can be extremely difficult to do and may not be practical in all cases. I had to strike a compromise, providing shelter and food but not much else.

Giving the addicted daughter time to "think about it" or "get ready" can lead not only to her disappearing back into abuse, it can also resurrect the walls of denial and other defenses that are a parent's way of handling pain and the shame of stigma. Therefore, a planned intervention aims at getting the addict into treatment immediately afterward if she agrees to go. Rare is the addict or alcoholic who will pass up the chance for "one last high" if given any wriggle room. And that can sabotage the entire process. To maximize your chances of success take the following steps:

1. Research and plan the form the intervention will take. Decide who will be involved. It is wise not to include people she dislikes or a family member who could sabotage the meeting—that is, divert attention or turn it into a confrontation.

2. Research and prepare her treatment options (see Chapters Six and Seven).

3. Have her bag packed. Arrange for her to take a medical leave from school or job, if needed. The HIPAA Act (Health Insurance Portability and Accountability Act), ensures an

employer or college is bound to confidentiality and can't give access to her medical information without her express written consent. Under the Family and Medical Leave Act (FMLA) of 1993, an employee can't be fired if an employer finds out she is in rehab, as long as she requested the leave. (There are other laws that protect recovering addicts, notably the Americans with Disabilities Act, which considers people with addiction to be disabled and thereby entitled to "reasonable accommodation" by their employer.)

4. Have transportation ready.

Finding a Good Interventionist

Most treatment centers can help find a professional interventionist. You can also look into recommendations from others you know who have gone through the intervention process, or look on the website of The Association of Intervention Specialist Certification Board, which provides credentials of professional competency.

Questions to ask when evaluating a potential interventionist:

1. How long has he or she been doing interventions?
2. How does he or she conduct interventions?
3. Do you feel you can be totally honest with this person?
4. Does this interventionist's approach make sense to you?
5. What does it cost? (see below)
6. Are you ready to commit to the process?

How Much Does an Intervention Cost?

A formal intervention is a financial investment, and it is not cheap. Rates can vary widely—I've seen quotes from $2,500 to $10,000. If the professional has to fly to your home, the costs include roundtrip airline tickets and lodging fees, plus incidentals. And, if need be, there's the cost of transporting your daughter to a recovery center. Health insurance coverage currently does not include interventions, but certain rehabilitation facilities offer low-cost loan programs that help not only to finance a stay in rehabilitation but also intervention and related travel expenses.

After the Intervention

If the intervention (including the informal, free type I used with my daughter) is successful in that your daughter agrees to get help, she'll typically go first to a detoxification center, or "detox," for at least three to five or seven days, where she will be medically monitored and given a physical work-up. A well-known addiction psychiatrist warns against simply sending an addict to a hospital and then discharging him or her without further treatment.[6] Why? Because addicts will be in a vulnerable physical state: their system has been cleansed of the heavy load of substances. Because they are now "clean," even a much smaller amount of the same drug they used heavily before can lead to an overdose. So a detoxed addict without some form of support or treatment has few defenses against cravings, and is strongly advised to enter some form of treatment upon discharge from detox. When in inpatient treatment, there will be a seamless move to safe, monitored quarters.

If Intervention Doesn't Succeed

Even if your daughter refuses to recognize she has a problem and to get treatment, know the intervention has accomplished something important: you have now changed the dynamic. You've let her know with loving concern what you expect of her, and you've been clear about the consequences of her refusal.

There are other steps you can take. You can seek family counseling. A family therapist is specifically trained to guide conversations to help resolve issues and develop communication, not least of which for marriages that come under such strain during a child's addiction. Sources of referrals include physicians, counselors, social workers, psychologists, and marriage and family therapists, all of whom have professional associations that can be located online.

Another option is seeking mediation conflict resolution, where a third party, trained in working with difficult situations and thinking "outside the box," assists the parent(s) and child to negotiate a settlement. If your daughter's situation is dire, you may also choose to get an involuntary commitment, where she is forced by the mental health system to enter inpatient care. This is a difficult procedure to enact wherein a treating psychiatrist must determine that inpatient treatment is needed. Another option is a court order, where the criminal justice system mandates legal consequences if treatment is refused. If the child is seventeen or younger, she is considered a juvenile and the records are usually expunged when she reaches twenty-one. If she is an adult, the criminal records will remain.

Remember despite any or all of these efforts, it may take your child a while to believe you are serious about getting her help to get well. Keep in mind she has a medically recognized brain disease, *not a moral weakness*. As a young alcoholic-addict, I wouldn't even consider I had a problem, despite the progressive loss of what I valued, even needed. It was only when all my safety nets were gone and a family member had a tough but loving talk with me that I began accepting the truth, and to ask for help. I had to get "sick and tired of being sick and tired." Know that for an addict this blessing of having to confront reality is a terrible feeling. To her it seems as if her life is over. Learning that she is not a bad person getting good, but a sick person getting well, is a huge revelation and can take time to absorb. Knowing there is a loving but firm family standing by can be a wonderful comfort and source of strength in early recovery.

Notes on Chapter Four

1. Anne Lamott, *Imperfect Birds: A Novel* (New York: Riverhead Books, 2011).

2. Dr. Jeffrey H. Samet, President of the American Board of Addiction Medicine, quoted in "Experts Call for Better Addiction Medicine Education for Physicians," Partnership for a Drug-Free Kids, October 25, 2013, http://www.drugfree.org/join-together/experts-call-for-better-addiction-medicine-education-for-physicians/.

3. George McGovern, *Terry: My Daughter's Life-and-Death Struggle with Alcoholism* (New York: Villard Books, 1995), 194.

4. See Robert J. Meyers and Brenda L. Wolfe, *Get Your Loved One Sober: Alternatives to Nagging, Pleading, and Threatening* (Center City, MN: Hazelden, 2004), xxii.

5. National Center on Addiction and Substance Abuse at Columbia University (CASA), June 2011, "Adolescent Substance Use: America's #1 Public Health Problem," http://www.casacolumbia.org/addiction-research/reports/adolescent-substance-use.

6. Adam Bisaga, Professor of Clinical Psychiatry at Columbia University College, in a community discussion hosted by Drug Crisis In Our Backyard (www.drugcrisisinourbackyard.com), Somers Middle School, New York, October 25, 2012.

Chapter Five

. . . .

Why Gender Matters in Substance Use Disorder

Increasing understanding of how men and women metabolize alcohol and other drugs differently, how they become addicted, and how gender affects recovery and relapse, is helping to reshape approaches to treatment. "Men and women exhibit structural and functional differences in key brain regions involved in drug addiction."[1] Yet the role of gender in substance use and abuse and recovery is a relatively new area of research. It wasn't until 1993 that the Federal Food and Drug Administration lifted a ban on testing women of child-bearing age in trials for drugs. Drugs were tested only or mostly on men, so scientists didn't know how they affect women until they were on the market. The dosage for the sleep medication Ambien, for example, which was tested on males, has been found recently to be twice as high as what is needed for females. For one thing, women have a higher percentage of body fat than men, and some drugs linger in the fat tissue, so the effects last longer.

The body-brain's systems of delivering the experiences of happiness, stress, coping, and dealing with pain are complex and highly calibrated. When potentially addictive substances enter this sensitive structure, the pathways of hormones and neurotransmitters (chemicals released by nerve cells to send signals to other nerve cells) are altered, and after repeated use, the brain needs the substance simply to avoid the pain and panic of withdrawal. The explanation of exactly what happens is a new frontier in science, a subject whose elegance and complexity we are just beginning to appreciate. We know the pathway of dopamine—the neurotransmitter responsible for reward-driven learning—is thought to be pathologically altered in addicted persons. Dr. Nora Volkow, a leading addiction expert, explains the physiology of addiction as boiling down to this: "The pleasure, pain, and devilish problem of control are simply the detritus left by waves of th[is] little molecule [dopamine] surging and retreating deep in the brain."[2]

Women have historically been underrepresented in clinical trials for many drugs, such as statins, for instance, for which there is little evidence of benefit to women, and they are still underrepresented in clinical trials of potential new drugs that are not government-funded. At least a partial explanation is the complications of gender hormones, what science calls the "estrous cycle," the phases of which can affect a test drug's efficacy, and must be factored into trials. Even more telling, "in the laboratory, gender bias in basic biomedical research and neuroscience is ingrained."[3] Even so, science is becoming clearer about the differences in the ways in which men and women addicts' brains ride those waves. For example, oxytocin is a stress-reducing hormone that promotes emotional bonding (and bonding, as we'll explore, is of particular importance in females). While women produce more oxytocin than men, chronic stress in addicted women produces prolonged secretion of another hormone called cortisol. This stress hormone lingers longer in women than in men, and in higher concentrations in addicted women, thus impeding the stress-reducer oxytocin. Not surprisingly, more cortisol is associated with symptoms of depression.

Estrogen, another sex hormone, is deficient in female addicts, which also adversely affects their sense of well-being. But that's just the start. Since the presence of estrogen enhances the neurotransmitter serotonin's receptivity in the female brain (serotonin levels affect a range of functions, including sexual desire, appetite, learning, and temperature regulation), less estrogen leads to lowered serotonin levels. And the presence or absence of estrogen also affects dopamine levels, which play a key role in mood. The bottom line here is addiction equals depression of the brain's major well-being chemicals in specific, significant ways for the female brain.

I have but skimmed the surface. A multitude of other chemicals at play in complex and particular ways in the female brain are adversely affected by addictive substances.[4] And as discussed previously, we can see why the progression to addiction appears to be accelerated in women.[5] Based on a cursory look at the function of key sex hormones and neurotransmitters, it is not surprising women are harder-hit, often at a younger age, by substance use disorders than men. Research is now teasing out the details of how this happens, such as the finding of one senior research scientist who determined the estrogenic hormone estradiol plays an important role in the increase of drug use in women, particularly during ovulation.[6]

Physiology, as well as brain chemistry, makes women vulnerable to addiction more quickly, with multiple kinds of damage. Why are two drinks for a woman who weighs, say, 140 pounds, equivalent to four to six drinks for a man of the same weight? As mentioned before, women's bodies have more fatty tissue than men's, and many drugs are absorbed more slowly in fat, so that a woman's brain and other organs are more exposed to them. Another complication occurs because women produce less of the stomach enzyme dehydrogenase, which breaks down alcohol in the digestive tract, leading to higher blood alcohol concentration. Because women's bodies hold on to alcohol and other drugs longer, they deteriorate faster than men. In plain language, a woman will tend to get drunk or high faster, stay drunk or high longer, and get sicker faster than a man her size. Of course, addiction wreaks havoc on men as well, yet it is clear that women addicts are at greater risk of more quickly becoming susceptible to a host of related ailments than their male counterparts.

Moderate drinking—one drink a day for women—can have health benefits. But heavy using can adversely affect women's bodies in the following ways:

Liver injury—Because chemicals take longer to pass through the higher amounts of fatty tissue in a woman's liver, a female is more likely to develop inflammation of the liver (hepatitis), and to die from cirrhosis, a consequence of chronic liver disease leading to loss of liver function. Combining alcohol with estrogen appears to increase the risk of liver damage.

Osteoporosis—This disease of the bones leads to an increased risk of bone loss and fracture. After menopause, bone mass is lost rapidly. Even small amounts of alcohol cause the body to excrete calcium, a mineral that aids in the decrease of the rate of fractures.

Digestive and nutritional problems—In the later stages of addiction, women suffer malnutrition and anemia much faster than men.

Heart disease and stroke—Heavy drinking can cause high blood fats (triglycerides), which can lead to becoming at risk for heart attacks and strokes due to atherosclerosis (narrowing of the arteries with a buildup of fatty plaques), as well as fatty liver disease, diabetes, kidney disease, and pancreatitis (inflammation of the pancreas that requires immediate medical attention).

High blood pressure—Also known as hypertension, high blood pressure puts a strain on blood vessels throughout the body and brain and can also lead to stroke, heart attack, or kidney disease.

Cancer—Alcoholism is a known contributor to cancers of the mouth, throat, voice box, esophagus, liver, colon, and rectum, and may increase the risk of pancreatic cancer. For women, the risk of breast cancer goes up due to increased estrogen production. Research continues to show that drinking alcohol increases a woman's risk of hormone-receptor-positive breast cancer and also that it increases breast cancer risk by damaging cell DNA.[7]

Impairment of the endocrine system—In this system of glands, each secretes different hormones into the bloodstream to help regulate such functions as metabolism, growth, development, tissue function, and mood.

Ob-gyn problems—Fertility may be affected as a result of substance use disorder, which may also contribute to early menopause, increased problems in pregnancy, and a range of negative effects on newborn children.

Weakened immune system—Chronic heavy drinking by women leads to less ability to fight infections and tumors because estrogen levels, beneficial to the immune system, are depressed. For both women and men, heavy drinking can also raise steroidal hormones (glucocorticoids), which suppress immune responses.

Brain damage—Women who drink excessively may be more vulnerable than men, and more quickly, to experience alcohol-induced brain damage such as atrophy (shrinkage) of the brain and memory loss.

Shortened lifespan—The female alcoholic is more likely to die prematurely because of alcohol-contributed diseases.[8]

That the body and brain of an addicted woman are impacted in devastating ways is not the end of the story. Substance use disorder would be simpler to treat if it were a brain/body disease, like, say, diabetes. Yet it is more than that. One expert, Dr. James West, calls addiction a "bio-psycho-spiritual-socio disease."[9]

Let's look at the tangled web addiction makes of female identity and her sense of self-worth. In an acclaimed memoir, Carolyn Knapp considered the way her drinking interfered with "the larger, murkier business of identity difficult enough for everyone, but particularly difficult for women and . . . close to impossible for women who drink."[10] The same holds true for those addicted to substances other than alcohol.

The way women form a sense of self has long been thought to occur in the same way as it does for men. Just as there was (and still is) reluctance in the "hard" sciences to test drugs on females, a similar bias exists in the social sciences. One stunning example: The eminent psychologist Erik Erikson developed a theory about identity in the late 1950s that gained widespread acceptance. After lengthy studies, he theorized that the developmental goal for children is autonomy, meaning independence and self-sufficiency. Erikson did not include girls in his studies! Emerging research strongly indicates a big gender difference in the development of children. "Girls define themselves not, as Erikson believed . . .[but] by their relationships with friends and family"[11] or, to put it another way, by moving toward connectedness with others. New research shows that when a woman's close relationship is severed or damaged, certain neurochemicals that promote well-being—serotonin, dopamine, and the bonding chemical oxytocin—take a nose dive, and cortisol, the stress hormone, surges. The result is anxiety, loneliness, and a sense of rejection.[12] The neurochemical balance of a woman struggling with addiction is already skewed by her addiction, and it is damaged even more intensely by the loss of connection. For a woman who is trying to recover, how she learns to handle feelings of rejection, loneliness, and social isolation play a significant part in her success at recovery.

This newer model in which girls' social development is characterized far more by connectedness than autonomy is reinforced by recent research on the "fight-or-flight" theory that has long been accepted as the model for the way people respond to high stress—that is, with aggression or withdrawal. Yet it turns out this model was developed by exclusively evaluating males. The hormone testosterone is associated with aggression and the "fight" response, and yes, women produce it too—but about ten times less so than men. Recent studies that focus solely on women's response to stress show another pattern, called the tend-and-befriend model. According to Dr. Leonard Sax, "We now know that females are wired to respond to stress in a different way than males are . . . Girls tend to want to be friends when under stress" [whereas boys tend to] "want to be alone." Other researchers into gender differences add "boys not only have less serotonin than girls have, but they also have less oxytocin, the primary human bonding chemical."[13]

During a highly significant period of stress, such as admitting she has a substance use problem and needs help to stop using and get well, a woman confronted by what the twelve-step fellowships call "the wreckage of our past" is in a vulnerable state, typically cut off from the sources of nurture and interaction she would have if she were healthy. Since the stress-related hormone cortisol lingers longer in women than in men, it is more difficult for females to let go of emotional turmoil, and they are more likely to experience anxiety and a weakening of their immune systems.

During adolescence, when both girls and boys are more likely to begin drinking or using drugs than at any other age, girls tend to be antisocial and secretive when courting risky behavior. Boys respond to risk and danger differently. They are more likely to seek out risky situations just for the sake of living dangerously.[14] Girls, on the other hand, may turn in on themselves, drinking or drugging, and/or using other self-harming behaviors. Often related to issues with body image, these can be eating disorders, cutting, and unprotected sex, with about twice the rate of sexually transmitted diseases as men, including HIV/AIDS.

Woven through women's experiences with substance use disorder and self-harm is the red thread of shame. "As women, our experiences were vastly different from men's," writes recovered alcoholic Jennifer Storm. "We walked around with shame and guilt that ate at the very core of our beings"[15]—shame, guilt, trauma, depression. Shame about being an alcoholic or addict, shame about being a woman who is addicted, shame about being an addicted mother, betraying the parent-child bond.

Of course men also suffer shame, guilt, and depression. But young women have a significantly higher rate of underlying depression than young men. Suicide attempts are more common among the total female population than males and much more common among female alcoholics. Male depression is often secondary to substance use and remits after he gets into recovery. (Exceptions are those who have a co-existing mental disorder, such as bipolar disorder.)

A crucial part of helping a young woman with substance use disorder and/or self-harm and mental health problems is recognizing she may be dealing with shame—and often, with trauma. As much as a parent doesn't want to "go there," it is a reality that many women substance users have suffered some sort of abuse—physical, sexual, or emotional—frequently resulting in trauma, which may present as depression or post-traumatic stress disorder (PTSD). We need to know that one out of every four girls will be sexually abused before the age of fourteen.[16]

When I was using, the moment I started thinking about an attack I'd experienced, I became anxious and hyper-aware. Research has found that trauma can change brain chemistry, just as substance abuse can change brain chemistry. I began to heal from my frightening experience only after I joined my twelve-step group and eventually went into therapy.

"What the research shows," a director at a top-ranked recovery center told me "is that men can get through their trauma, and move on. But women don't want to revisit the trauma. Women can hang on to trauma forever and it is a trigger [for relapse]."[17] When we consider the way hormones and neurotransmitters operate in the female brain (the lingering cortisol stress hormone), this makes sense. Experts in addiction treatment and researchers who focus on women emphasize also that young women appear to particularly benefit from longer treatment. At the Betty Ford Center's young adult program for ages eighteen to twenty-five, for example, females are required to be in treatment twice as long as males because "experience and research," states an extensive survey, "substantiate that a high percentage of female addicts suffer significant trauma."[18] Professionals agree longer treatment for addiction is important but, as anyone who deals with health insurance companies knows, it's not available at this time. Insurance company actuaries continue to fend off the clear need for more than a few weeks of treatment for women with addiction, particularly those who have co-existing disorders.

To summarize: Differing hormones affect the way women and men respond to stress, as do psychological and sociological differences. These distinctions affect women and men differently both in terms of their addiction and in their recovery. Understanding these differences can have significant implications for applying the proper therapeutic techniques in dealing with both genders.

Other Mental and Emotional Issues
Impacting Women Substance Users

Emotional and mental problems can drive young women's addiction, even flourish during addiction, and such co-occurring disorders often drive her to use substances. I thought of myself as "looking for balance" when I was using drugs and alcohol. The umbrella term "stress" covers a wide range of mental conditions that impact addiction. More women than men opioid addicts have affective or mood disorders, anxiety, and major depression. Women are seven times more likely to have borderline personality disorders.[19] And women are twice as likely to have PTSD and four times more likely than men to develop PTSD when exposed to the same trauma."[20]

Ongoing Research on Women and Addiction

"For the most part," says Dr. Janine Austin Clayton, "looking for differences between males and females has been a blind spot in biomedical research, leaving gaps in our knowledge."[21] Among recent research projects about addiction and gender is a study that measures the serotonin system's much faster damage in the brains of female versus male alcoholics. The function of alcoholic women's serotonin system may fall by 50 percent after four years, whereas it takes three times as long—twelve years—for the function of men's to be halved.[22]

Another important project currently underway is a National Institute on Drug Abuse (NIDA)-funded grant to design and pilot a new manual-based group therapy for women with substance use disorders. Shelly F. Greenfield, MD, a co-editor of *Women and Addiction* (The Guilford Press, 2009), is the principal investigator.

NIDA and The National Institute on Alcohol Abuse and Addiction (NIAAA) have large, ongoing research projects advancing the research on male-female differences in drug and alcohol abuse and addiction and on factors specific to women. Since 1995, NIDA has supported the Women and Sex/Gender Differences Research Program (WGRG) as a historically understudied area. It is coordinated by Dr. Cora Lee Wetherington. WGRG seeks to include new research tools and techniques—including new imaging modalities, molecular biology, and genetics—to identify and elucidate gender differences.

Several women-centered recovery centers have added "hormonal shift awareness therapy" to their treatment plans. Hormonal shift awareness therapy is based on the preliminary research of Donna Corrente, a clinical consultant and the former director of women's services at the Hanley Hazelden Treatment Center, and is designed to address women addicts' physical and emotional needs caused by the four hormonal stages of a woman's life: menstruation, peri-menopause, menopause, and post-menopause. The theory is that hormonal changes can "trigger" relapse in early recovery, particularly among women who are premenstrual—what my daughter complained about as "PMSing," or Premenstrual Syndrome. During fluctuations of the menstrual cycle, estrogen, the female sex hormone, interacts with endorphins in the brain to adversely affect levels of serotonin. When women's ovarian hormones are surging and cycling, the result can be moodiness, anxiety, anger, fatigue, and depression, leading to an increase in stress, another key element in addiction. Women in early recovery are also at greater risk of relapse due to an increased sensitivity to drugs resulting from their estrogen levels becoming elevated during active addiction. Remarkably, sensitivity to drugs remains even when the estrogen levels are reduced. The goal of hormonal shift awareness therapy is to educate women about what to expect during the four hormonal stages and how to mitigate these experiences naturally, using techniques such as yoga, meditation, visualization, deep breathing, and creative expression.[23]

In Chapter Six we'll discuss how such issues can be treated in gender-specific settings. Regardless of the setting, however, it is paramount that properly-trained professionals tease out and identify possible co-occurring disorders, be they of mood, personality, or cognition (thinking).

Notes on Chapter Five

1. Amanda Elton and Clinton D. Kilts, "The Roles of Sex Differences in the Drug Addiction Process," in *Women and Addiction: A Comprehensive Handbook*, edited by Sudie E. Back, Kathleen T. Brady, and Shelly F. Greenfield (New York: The Guilford Press, 2009), 163. Reprinted with permission.

2. Abigail Zuger, "A General in the Drug War," *The New York Times*, June 13, 2011. "General" Volkow pioneered the use of brain imaging in investigating the toxic effects and addictive properties of drugs.

3. Roni Caryn Rabin, "Labs Are Told to Start Including a Neglected Variable: Females," *The New York Times*, May 14, 2014.

4. For more see Louann Brizendine, *The Female Brain* (New York: Broadway Books, 2006).

5. Wendy J. Lynch, Marc N. Potenza, Kelly P. Cosgrove, and Carolyn M. Mazure, "Sex Differences in Vulnerability to Stimulant Abuse," in *Women and Addiction: A Comprehensive Handbook* edited by Kathleen T. Brady, Sudie E. Back, and Shelly F. Greenfield (New York: The Guilford Press, 2009), 414–15.

6. Jill B. Becker and Ming Hu, "Sex Differences in Drug Abuse," *Frontiers in Neuroendocrinology*, vol. 29, no. 1 (January 2008): 36–47, www.ncbi.nlm.nih.gov/pmc/articles/PMC2235192/, cited in Roni Caryn Rabin, "The Drug-Dose Gender Gap," *The New York Times*, May 15, 2014.

7. BreastCancer.org, November 13, 2013, "Drinking Alcohol," http://www.breastcancer.org/risk/factors/alcohol. See also National Center on Addiction and Substance Abuse at Columbia University (CASA), *Women Under the Influence* (Baltimore, MD: Johns Hopkins University Press, 2005), 68, citing a study that found women who drink two and a half to three drinks per day have a one-third increased risk of developing breast cancer compared to women who abstain.

8. Steven Reinberg, "Alcoholism Shortens Life more than Smoking: Study," *Healthday*, www.consumer.health/com.general-health-information-about-alcohol-abuse.

9. The Betty Ford Center, "BFC Pioneer Dr. James West, 93, Stays the Course," *Recovery News*, March 1, 2008, www.bettyfordcenter.org/recovery/recovery/bfc-pioneer-dr-james-west-93-stays-the-course.php.

10. Carolyn Knapp, *Drinking: A Love Story* (Los Angeles: The Dial Press, 1996), 74.

11. Cynthia Briggs and Jennifer Pepperell, *Women, Girls, and Addiction: Celebrating the Feminine in Counseling Treatment and Recovery* (New York: Routledge, 2009), 36.

12. See Brizendine, *The Female Brain*, 40.

13. Leonard Sax, *Why Gender Matters: What Parents and Teachers Need to Know about the Emerging Science of Sex Differences* (New York: Doubleday, 2005), 69, 83; and Michael Gurian and Kathy Stevens, "With Boys and Girls in Mind," *Educational Leadership* 62, no. 3 (November 2004): 21–26, http://www.ascd.org/publications/educational-leadership/nov04/vol62/num03/With-Boys-and-Girls-in-Mind.aspx.

14. Leonard Sax, *Why Gender Matters*, 41–42.

15. Jennifer Storm, *Blackout Girl: Growing Up and Drying Out in America* (Center City, MN: Hazelden 2008), 215.

16. James W. Hopper, *Child Sexual Abuse: Statistics, Research, Resources* (Boston: Boston University School of Medicine, 1998).

17. Conversation with Tom Deitzler, Director of the Young Adult Program at The Caron Center for Recovery, 2010.

18. D. D. Simpson and P. M. Flynn, "Drug Abuse Treatment Outcome Studies (DATOS): A National Evaluation of Treatment Effectiveness," *Encyclopedia of Substance Abuse Prevention, Treatment, and Recovery* (London and Thousand Oaks, CA: Sage Publishing, 2008), 303, 307.

19. Substance Abuse and Mental Health Services Administration (SAMHSA), "Medication-Assisted Treatment for Opioid Addiction in Opioid Treatment Programs," *Treatment Improvement Protocol (TIP)* Report 43 (Rockville, MD, 2005): 190–91.

20. Edna B. Ford, Terence M. Keane, et al., *Effective Treatment for PTSD* (The Guilford Press, 2009). Reprinted with permission.

21. Janine Austin Clayton, May 14, 2014, "Filling the Gaps: NIH to Enact New Policies to Address Sex Differences," *Office of Research on Women's Health at the National Institutes of Health*, http://orwh.od.nih.gov/about/director/director_nature_2014.asp.

22. Claudia Fahlke, et al., "Neuroendocrine Assessment of Serotonergic, Dopaminergic, and Noradrenergic Functions in Alcoholic Individuals," *Alcoholism: Clinical & Experimental Research* 36, no. 1 (January 2012): 97–103.

23. See "Hormone Therapy," website of The Orchid Recovery Center, http://www.orchidrecoverycenter.com/hormone-therapy.

Chapter Six

. . . .

Getting Her Effective Treatment

Sending a child to treatment is almost always a choice made out of desperation. It is also an incredible gift of hope.

If your daughter gets in trouble with the law as a result of her addiction, there may be an option through the courts in your community known as "Drug Court" or "Treatment Court." The offender is offered a contract that gives her access to treatment and health monitoring, sometimes through an outpatient facility or counseling service, sometimes with an additional component of community service. If she completes her treatment successfully, it can result in either suspension of her case or probation. Per the National Institute of Justice there are over 2,800 drug courts in the United States as of June 30, 2013.

There are also a number of alternatives to inpatient rehabilitation treatment for substance use disorder. One option is counseling, either individual and/or group. Check to ensure counselors have at least a master's degree before agreeing to this option. A second choice is outpatient treatment. This is helpful to some young people, but in our new world of opiate addiction, be advised that many are not yet able to handle the temptation of being in an environment where they know all the users and dealers and could easily relapse.

This was the case with my daughter and dozens of other young adults I have known personally, female and male. Many were finally able to stay in recovery only after they went to inpatient treatment centers with strong aftercare programs.

With the burgeoning use of drugs and the rising epidemic of heroin addiction, a larger number of women than ever before, including young women, are seeking treatment, although most still do not.[1] Still, according to one of the largest and oldest recovery centers, Hazelden—recently merged with the Betty Ford Center to become Hazelden Betty Ford Foundation—there has been a four-fold increase in admission inquiries from women in the last few years.

Getting effective treatment for your daughter is not easy, partly because of what addiction medicine specialists have called "a disconnect" with mainstream medical practice. As of this writing, no national standards of care have been implemented for treatment facilities for addiction, although the national Substance Abuse and Mental Health Services Administration (SAMHSA) is working toward that goal. Meanwhile, "patients face a patchwork of treatment programs with vastly different approaches."[2] As one parent describes it: "If a kid really has a problem, where is [s]he going to get treatment? I found myself in this position, and I'm an expert in the field. I had no idea. If I wanted to buy a refrigerator, I'd go to Consumer Reports and get information. So why don't we make a Consumer Reports for substance abuse programs?"[3] What is a parent to do? If we need surgery or have cancer, we are not asked to become experts. Most of us will do basic research and rely on the medical establishment to treat what ails us. But when we're looking for addiction treatment for our children or ourselves, the same standard doesn't apply. When I knew my daughter needed treatment, rather than going to my beloved family doctor who is great at treating aches and pains but not an expert on addiction, I reached out first to other parents of children who suffered from addiction. I got a lot of conflicting, anecdotal suggestions. It was through that chance conversation in a bank that I learned about a recovery center that had proven success in treating women, and particularly younger women. (I will discuss the various approaches and benefits of effective gender-specific treatment in Chapter Seven.) To increase your odds of success, know what to look for in a facility.

How Do You Know Whether the Treatment Facility Is Effective?

It can be a challenge to find out whether a particular center actually delivers on what it promises. How can you measure the validity of claims and testimonials posted on their websites, in television ads, or even made by their staff during interviews?

Here are some key factors to look out for

* a proven treatment modality that uses evidence-based care;
* adherence to medical standards;
* a program that addresses the underlying issues of addiction;
* a family component;
* good aftercare and relapse prevention strategies.

I will provide you with clear explanations and examples of each of these key factors here and in the following chapter.

Licensing and Accreditation: Helpful Tools

You will want to know, first and foremost, how successful a rehabilitation center is in helping their patients get into recovery—and stay in recovery. Useful statistics are hard to come by despite a growing chorus of complaints. I found few solid statistics about the percentage of clients who stayed in a program and remained in recovery afterward.

To date, there is no requirement for facilities to keep uniform statistics that can be evaluated by the public. "It is shocking," declares one doctor who treats addiction, "how few drug treatment programs can even offer complete reliable statistics. . . . There is no incentive, no requirement, for any program to keep figures, let alone release them to the public, and without the facts there is no reason to admit to anything but success."[4] Practically speaking, it can of course be difficult to keep track of people once they leave a treatment center, especially long-term. Furthermore, most rehab centers do not share their methodology in tracking "outcomes," and resist sharing information about how they work, according to long-time treatment expert A. Thomas McLellan, Executive Director of the Treatment Research Institute. Its Center on Policy Research and Analysis helps states and local governments develop and evaluate evidence-based policies within existing budgets.

What it comes down to is this: most "evidence" about rehabs is anecdotal. Evidence from studies in the field suggests a 30 percent success rate one year after treatment is considered good. This correlates with surveys Alcoholics Anonymous conducts of members every few years. Its most recently-released study reported 33 percent were sober more than ten years; 12 percent for five to ten years; 24 percent one to five years; and 31 percent less than a year.[5] A well-regarded Stanford University study reported that at sixteen years after they stopped using, people who participated in twelve-step groups had a thirty-three percent higher success rate than non-participants.[6] Other studies point to similar efficacy for recovery among Cognitive Behavioral Therapy (CBT), Motivational Enhancement Therapy, and twelve-step programs. But while there is no magic bullet when it comes to recovery from addiction, parents armed with the right questions and knowledge are in the best position to help their children.

There is much new research aimed at understanding how to arrest addiction and promote long-term recovery. A five-year comprehensive research study at the Hanley Center (now an Origins Recovery Center) isolated and tracked how each therapeutic action with each patient, from admission to rehabilitation, at 30, 90, 180, 270, and 360 days, impacted the indicators of recovery. The results were published in 2013 and suggest, among other things, that limiting interventions to spirituality, CBT, relapse prevention, and social support would yield significant benefits, as well as paying special attention to Baby Boomers, Generation Xers, and women.[7]

In the meantime, know that each state has licensing requirements for quality standards compliance at addiction treatment centers. Also, each state has its own office pertaining to alcoholism and drug abuse. In my own state of New York, the New York State Office of Alcoholism and Substance Abuse Services (OASAS.ny.gov) provides extensive information about the various applicable laws and regulations. Some states have recently improved the accountability process, such as assessing how effectively programs work for clients if they're state-funded. Oregon, for one, mandates programs use evidence-based practices, techniques that have been shown to be effective in studies. But every state has different requirements, so check those in yours. Furthermore, facilities that receive federal funding (via the Substance Abuse Prevention and Treatment Block Grant) must meet grant requirements: The US Department of Health and Human Services provides a list of those treatment centers. An online publication by the National Institute on Drug Abuse called "Seeking Drug Abuse Treatment: Know What to Ask" helps refine the search.

All prospective recovery centers can be checked for accreditation. The organization CARF International (Commission on Accreditation of Rehabilitation Facilities) is an independent, nonprofit accreditor of health and human services facilities throughout the world since 1966. CARF-accredited providers "conform to proven business practices and commit to continuous quality improvements."[8] Another organization, the National Association of Addiction Treatment Providers (NAATP.org), founded in 1978, represents about 275 not-for-profit and for-profit treatment providers. Per their mission statement, they are committed to providing "leadership, advocacy, training, and other member support services to assure the continued availability and highest quality of addiction treatment."

Understanding Treatment Options

Before entering any program of recovery, medically supervised detoxification is frequently recommended. Detoxification, or detox, is the process of the body ridding itself of a drug or drugs. Many addicts are so fearful of the pain of withdrawal that they continue to use substances even when they don't want to. Indeed, in the old days, detox usually meant going "cold turkey," often at home. Today, medical detox programs should closely monitor alcohol and other drug withdrawal, which can have dangerous and even life-threatening consequences. They should also take into account the unique characteristics of each patient's health and addiction. Detox is not treatment, but it prepares the individual for the next step in the treatment she needs.

Once a patient is detoxified from opiates, he or she will often be given drug blockers. Treatment providers remain divided on whether blockers in early recovery improve rates of recovery. When the venerable Hazelden Center added medicine therapy (Medication Assisted Treatment or MAT) to its program in 2013 in response to the growing number of young opiate addicts seen in rehabs, it was taken as a strong signal that evidence-based therapy is now mainstream.[9] Physicians who specialize in addiction medicine promote judicious use of agonists and partial agonists, blockers, and other medications for substance abuse and co-occurring disorders, such as depression and bipolar disorder, as a way to increase the odds of addicts completing treatment and staying in recovery.

Drugs that help addicts avoid using opiates include:

- Naltrexone. An opioid antagonist used to help treat alcohol cravings as well as long-term opioid dependence. Chemically, it is similar to Naloxone; however, Naloxone is used primarily in the emergency settings to reverse the acute effects of opiates and opioids.
- Buprenorphine. Known by the brand names Suboxone and Subutex, it is a semi-synthetic opioid that works as a "partial agonist" to help block the ability to get high from other opioids.
- Methadone. A synthetic opioid that works as a "full agonist" and is used to manage withdrawal symptoms and reduce opioid dependency, and comes under many brand names, including Dolophine, Methadose, and Diskets.
- LAAM (Levo-Alpha-Acetylmethadol). Used as a "second-line" treatment, when opioid dependent individuals have failed to respond to other agents.

Research into creating a vaccine to immunize against heroin is underway, though scientists say federal spending on drug-addiction research is still a low priority for the government. Other researchers are studying the genetics of addiction to find which genes make people more susceptible to addiction, as well as testing an opioid that dissolves in the stomach and is not addictive that could be used to treat opiate addicts in the future.

While a growing number of physicians and addiction scientists are convinced using such medicines in conjunction with treatment gives addicts a better chance at maintaining recovery, the treatment community as a whole is by no means in agreement. Some argue for short-term use of medical aids, while others opt for a residential inpatient treatment and peer-support system with complete abstinence. Others, such as Mark Willenberg, MD, former director of treatment and recovery research at the National Institute for Alcohol Abuse and Alcoholism, counter that the drugs used to block addiction aren't the problem; it's the doctors who don't know how to use them. Many treatment programs lag behind the science. A recent national survey of opioid treatment programs found only 8 to 9 percent of all facilities offered medication-assisted therapy.[10] Reflecting this controversy, there is a wide range of opinions among members of twelve-step groups on the use of various prescribed medications in aid of a member's recovery and mental health.

Suboxone was an important aid in supporting my daughter's early, tentative recovery from opiate addiction. Kim was regularly monitored by the doctors who prescribed it and gradually "tapered off" to the lowest possible dosage, at which time she went through an uncomfortable but manageable near-week of withdrawal symptoms that resembled the flu. She views her commitment to recovery as the crucial component, not the use of Suboxone. And she points out addicts sometimes sell Suboxone to obtain their drug of choice, and while it doesn't provide a "high," Suboxone is an opioid and therefore causes dependency. If nothing else, using it or other blockers has kept addicts from resorting to the use of "street" drugs, and at its best, has helped thousands of addicts wean themselves off prescription painkillers and heroin. While there is disagreement about the use of Suboxone among twelve-step fellowships, many do agree "medications are an important part of treatment for many patients, especially when combined with counseling and other behavioral therapies."[11]

Here are some of the main evidence-based behavioral and psychosocial therapies recommended in treatment:

- Cognitive Behavioral Therapy (CBT). Teaches the client to identify situations that put her at high risk, to develop strategies for handling specific situations, and to learn to identify and cope with cravings. One study showed significantly fewer female clients with PTSD dropped out of CBT than problem-solving therapy.[12]

- Motivational Enhancement Therapy (MET). Motivates the client to change her behavior via her own resources.
- Dialectical Behavioral Therapy (DBT). Combines CBT techniques with concepts of mindful awareness—a modality drawn from contemplative practices, including meditation, yoga, art, and spending time in nature. Research over the last decade shows mindfulness helps foster well-being in many ways, including alleviating anxiety and depression.
- Group therapy. Helps patients come to terms with the harmful consequences of their drug use disorder and boosts their motivation to stay drug free.

Other types and approaches to treatment are often used in combination in therapeutic communities (TCs):

- Fostering personal and social responsibility via peer influence and group therapy, self-help, and "mutual self-help" (recommended especially for young adults).
- Attendance at twelve-step meetings.
- Faith-based approaches.
- Wilderness treatments.

Other techniques include acupuncture, hypnosis, Eye Movement Desensitization and Reprocessing (EMDR) for post-traumatic stress disorder (PTSD), Native American customs, and more. On some techniques the jury is still out. For example, although some therapists swear by it, the evidence for EMDR's effectiveness is inconclusive.[13] Nor is there sufficient evidence for the efficacy of Craniosacral Therapy (CST), a bodywork technique that aims at regulating the flow of cerebrospinal fluid through light therapeutic touch, which is said to dissipate negative emotional experiences.

To be effective, a recovery program must target an individual's unique needs with the proper professional expertise. Co-occurring disorders (such as addiction and depression) as well as multiple manifestations of addiction often occur in young women. Other disorders young women struggle with include self-harm, such as cutting, anxiety, bipolar disorder, or untreated ADHD. Counselors should be specifically trained to deal with such disorders.

Regardless of the diagnosis, many studies show relapse rates drop steadily the longer an addict stays in treatment.[14]

Questions to Ask a Recovery Center

- Is the program run by state-accredited, licensed, and/or trained professionals?
- Is the facility clean, organized, and well-run? If you can't look at a place in person, ask for references and call them.
- Does the program encompass the full range of needs of my loved one—medical (including treatment of infectious diseases); psychological (including any co-occurring mental illness); social; vocational; legal?
- Does the facility specialize in treating addiction to the substance/s my child is taking? For example, if your child is addicted to one of the new synthetic substances such as bath salts, opiates, or methamphetamines, each of these needs a distinct regimen of detoxification. For instance, treatment for methamphetamine addiction may need to occur at a center specializing in the psychoses that can result from meth use.
- If applicable to your situation, does the program also address sexual orientation? Physical disabilities? Does it provide age-, gender-, and culturally-appropriate treatment services?
- Is there ongoing assessment of my child's treatment plan to ensure it meets her changing needs?
- Does the program employ strategies to engage and keep individuals in longer-term treatment, increasing the likelihood of success?
- Does the program offer counseling (individual or group) and other behavioral therapies? What kind of behavioral therapies?
- Does it offer medication as part of the treatment regimen, if appropriate?
- Is long-term aftercare support and/or guidance encouraged, provided, or maintained?
- What are the procedures in case my daughter breaks the rules or relapses?

- Are services or referrals offered to family members? What are they?
- Can you speak to other parents or their children who have been at the facility?

What to Expect While Your Daughter Is in Treatment

Once you've decided on a recovery center and enrolled your daughter, what happens next? This can be a time of relief. She is in a safe place where she'll hopefully learn to break bad habits and relationships and acquire healthy new attitudes. Yet, as her parent, it's hard to be away from her during this difficult time. You should be able to talk to the staff and doctors at the facility often. They'll help determine the length of her stay, advise you about finances, and any other concerns you may have. If the counselor assigned to your daughter doesn't call you within the first few days of treatment, call and initiate a dialogue.

After medical detox, your daughter will be assigned a clinical team, including a counselor, who will work together for and with her throughout her time at the treatment center. If she is assessed with a dual diagnosis—such as an anxiety disorder, depression, or bipolar disorder in addition to her chemical dependency—it is important both conditions be treated.

Your child's recovery will mostly occur in group interactions, but she will also have individual counseling. Her treatment should include good nutrition, physical activities, and some type of spiritual exercises (yoga, meditation, prayer). Recreation—learning how to have fun in recovery—should also be included in her regimen. Finally, an aftercare (or step-down) plan should be developed for her, whether it be a sober living facility, ongoing counseling, and/or encouragement to continue participating in twelve-step programs or other mutual support recovery groups.

If your daughter is over eighteen, she is legally entitled to refuse to give the staff permission to talk with you. However, the best recovery centers stress and encourage family involvement; some even require it. To the fullest extent you can, be involved in your daughter's recovery. While most rehab centers do not allow the use of cell phones, laptops, and other wireless devices (they are distractions and allow clients to stay in touch with bad influences), some centers will allow access to phones and supervised Internet use later on in the recovery process. If she won't talk to you, write her letters.

If your daughter does call to complain about the recovery center (she's not getting anything out of it . . . the food is bad . . . she hates the place), talk to the counselor. Keep in mind manipulation is part and parcel of an addict's mindset and is not something that changes overnight.

If she allows you to visit and you are able to do so, visit her and talk with her clinical team. This will be a good time to talk to the team and then to your child about your "bottom lines," such as what you will and will not allow after treatment. For example, if you will allow your daughter to live at home after treatment, what are your conditions? If she does not allow you to visit, then read her your "bottom-line" letter over the phone, or send it by mail.

In setting your boundaries, be encouraging and supportive. Let her know how proud you are of the steps she has taken to deal with her problem. Be firm and offer concrete suggestions if she's unhappy with the program she's in. You could suggest going to another inpatient or outpatient program; seeing a counselor; and/or attending mutual support recovery meetings.

Support her, but do not enable: you may decide to offer support after rehab—use of a car, money—but be clear this will be conditional on her adhering to your terms (such as being monitored to stay in recovery, getting a job, or going to school).

A friend of mine temporarily took in her nephew when he was released from rehab because the young man had nowhere else to go. As a condition of living in her house, he had to attend either one twelve-step meeting a week or see a therapist. When he balked, she held firm. Reluctantly, he agreed to go to a meeting and ended up making new friends who became a good support network in his recovery.

Have a backup plan in the event she insists on leaving the treatment facility early. Consult with her clinical team for guidance. If she has reached the age of eighteen, she has the legal right to leave, but if your child is younger and she runs away from her treatment center or your home, you can seek intervention from the legal system. There are a number of resources to help find her (see the Appendix). You may also want to hire an attorney who specializes in juvenile justice.

Paying for Rehab

Getting into recovery always makes financial sense, despite the costs. Think of the money that has been squandered on alcohol and other drugs, on counseling, legal bills, or healthcare—and the mounting costs to your child's physical and mental health. My own epiphany about the costs occurred when I found out Kim had sold the car she'd been given by her father to a drug dealer. Since I was the title holder, I received hundreds of dollars in parking tickets until I finally declared the car abandoned. This was a costly lesson for me—one of several. However you cut it, addiction is expensive, for everyone concerned. And getting well is an investment in her future.

The Least-to-Most-Expensive Forms of Treatment

- *Outpatient.* The patient attends several weekly sessions at a local facility.
- *Partial (PHP).* The patient attends half-day sessions at a local facility.
- *State or federally-funded inpatient (residential) facility.* Accepts health insurance, including Medicare.
- *Private inpatient facility.* Some accept health insurance, others accept partial-pay health insurance, some are self-pay. Costs range from about $400 to $2,000 a day.

As of 2014, the Affordable Care Act requires all small group and individual market plans created before March 23, 2010, to comply with Federal parity requirements, enacted in the Mental Health Parity and Addiction Equity Act (MHPAEA). This means the Health Insurance Marketplaces in every state must include coverage for mental health and substance use disorders as one of ten categories of essential health benefits, and the coverage must comply with MHPAEA.[15] Effective as of 2014, Medicaid is now based on income, up to 133 percent of the federal poverty level, and not disability, increasing access to services for substance use and mental disorders. People whose income exceeds the limit for Medicaid can access healthcare via state or federal health insurance exchanges. As a result of healthcare reform millions of people who need treatment (including 80 to

90 percent of people with substance abuse disorder) may now be able to get treatment because mental health, behavioral, and substance abuse treatment is now mandatory for certain periods. There are two downsides, however:

1) Only outpatient care is mandated, and insurers often refuse to cover inpatient care unless and until an individual has failed to enter or maintain recovery through an outpatient program.

2) There is a shortage of providers and available beds to accommodate the influx of the newly-insured who need treatment.

Find out how much treatment costs, and ask about any possible additional expenses at the program or facility you have chosen for your daughter's care. Find out from your insurer what your copayments and deductibles are. Be prepared to stand up for your rights. The good news is legal access to care for substance abuse has evolved; however, some health insurance providers can limit which rehab facilities you may choose. If you are limited by your insurance to one choice, research that facility. If you don't think it would be a good placement for your loved one, find out how you can contest the referral.

Again, many experts with long-term experience in the field of addiction treatment concur a short-term stay—often with a twenty-eight to thirty-day limit on inpatient treatment—is demonstrably insufficient, and they argue for longer care. Several rehabilitation centers now even mandate a ninety-day stay. Few public or private insurance programs currently authorize longer treatment, but some will have degrees of flexibility. Talk to a prospective rehab center about scholarships and financial assistance grants, sliding scale fees, and/or payment plans. The center may offer either an in-house financing program with affordable and flexible credit terms or work with external medical financing companies that lend part or all of the cost with longer-term payments. I and many parents I've talked to have found that good centers want to work with you to help your child. Assistance programs to help offset medical costs may also be available via social service organizations at your local or state level.

If you have good credit and are confident you will be able to make the loan payments, you may want to look into a healthcare or medical credit card. Available from care providers, such cards are used exclusively for medical expenses (prescriptions, surgeries, and insurance deductibles).

It is a loan that allows you to buy your child the treatment she needs but can't afford. If you can't make scheduled payments, however, you may incur large penalties and much higher interest rates. So if you are financially burdened or uncertain about your ability to make payments, this is probably not a wise option for you. Another way to raise funds is to sell a large-ticket item, such as a car or expensive jewelry, or to refinance a home to cover the cost of your loved one's treatment. Some people turn to family members for assistance.

Sending your child to a recovery center is a significant financial investment. As with all investments, it comes with risks. Just because a student graduates from college, for example, doesn't guarantee she'll find a good job. Our hope has to be that "graduation" from rehab will mean health, long-term recovery, and self-responsibility; however, my own daughter is an all-too-common example of how it can go the other way, too. When Kim went into her first rehab she "talked the talk" alright, but she didn't "walk the walk." Within a year, she was in rehab again, but this time far away from her network of user-friends and dealers, in a recovery community of other women, and then in a sober living house. Eventually she started drinking briefly and then went back to heroin again, stopping and starting on her own until she became a committed member of two twelve-step fellowships and received the right medication for her depression.

Parents don't want to hear stories about how relapse is part of the process of recovery. I sure didn't. When a counselor at Kim's first recovery place told me gently that young people often don't "make it" the first time, I was furious and terrified. I thought, *Isn't it their job to get them to quit using?* Even so, I did know from my own experience that it is the job of the addict to get well. That what looks like failure can turn out to be progress. Remembering addiction is driven by a powerful mental obsession and a physical compulsion, "failure"—what twelve-step groups call "picking up" and "going back out," and what the medical community calls "relapse"— can often turn out to be steps on the road toward achieving health. Even if she resumes using, a new foundation has been laid. As Kim shared with me recently, what she had learned by being in a community of women working to overcome their addiction in positive, nurturing ways, stayed with her after she relapsed. She remembered how the shame and guilt lifted during her period of living in recovery with other women, and how much she enjoyed simple things like eating in a restaurant, playing sports, and, yes, interacting with young men who attended twelve-step meetings. She had learned she was not a bad person trying to get good, but a sick person trying to get well. The seed of the idea of living a full, happy life, without alcohol and other drugs, had been planted. Thousands of young women do recover after false starts.

Implications for Treatment Related to the Affordable Care Act

Many experts think we are at a crossroads with treatment options for our addicted loves ones. The Affordable Care Act's provisions for including substance abuse treatment as part of healthcare coupled with the escalating drug use epidemic in our country are creating an urgent demand for more services. According to Peter Luongo, Executive Director of the Institute for Research, Education & Training in Addictions, "If you're going to have a health system of primary care that you pay for to keep people well, you can't do that if people have undiagnosed, untreated substance abuse disorders."[16]

Notes on Chapter Six

1. Addiction Treatment Forum (online), "Seeking and Getting Substance Abuse Treatment: Barriers Women Face," April 21, 2013, http://atforum.com/2013/04/seeking-and-getting-substance-abuse-treatment-barriers-women-face/.

2. National Center on Addiction and Substance Abuse at Columbia University (CASA), June 2012, "Addiction Medicine," ii, http://www.casacolumbia.org/addiction-research/reports/addiction-medicine.

3. Dr. A. Thomas McLellan, quoted in Felicia D'Ambrosio, "Q&A with Dr. A. Thomas McLellan, Director of the Treatment Research Institute," April 3, 2012, http://www.generocity.org/qa-with-dr-a-thomas-mclellan-director-of-the-treatment-research-institute/.

4. Michael Stein, *The Addict: One Patient, One Doctor, One Year* (New York: Harper Perennial, 2010), 17–18.

5. Kevin Gray, "Does A.A. Really Work? A Round-Up of Recent Studies," *The Fix*, January 29, 2012, http://www.thefix.com/content/the-real-statistics-of-aa7301.

6. Rudolf H. Moos and Bernice S. Moos, "Treated and Untreated Alcohol-Use Disorders: Course and Predictors of Remission and Relapse," *Evaluation Review* 31, no. 6 (December 2007): 564–84.

7. Karen Dodge, PhD; Barbara Krantz, DO, MS; Paul J. Kenny, PhD; and Gabriel P. Suciu, PhD, "Substance Abuse Treatment Modalities and Outcomes in a Naturalistic Setting," *Addictive Disorders & Their Treatment* 12, no. 2 (June 2013): 76–90.

8. Commission on Accreditation of Rehabilitation Facilities (CARF), "The public says: Accreditation Matters!," http://www.carf.org/Public/.

9. Maia Szalavitz, "Hazelden Introduces Antiaddiction Medications into Recovery for First Time," Time.com, November 5, 2012, www.healthland.time.com/2012/11/05.

10. Substance Abuse and Mental Health Services Administration (SAMHSA), "National Survey of Substance Abuse Treatment Services, 2011," quoted in Jane Brody, "Effective Addiction Treatment," *The New York Times*, February 6, 2013.

11. National Institute on Drug Abuse (NIDA), "Seeking Drug Abuse Treatment: Know What to Ask," (last updated June 2013), www.drugabuse.gov/publications/seeking-drug-abuse-treatment-know-what-to-ask.

12. Annemarie McDonagh, et al., "Randomized Trial of Cognitive-Behavioral Therapy for Chronic PTSD in Adult Female Survivors of Childhood Sexual Abuse," *Journal of Consulting and Clinical Psychology* 73, no. 3 (June 2005): 515–24.

13. Scott Lilienfeld and Hal Arkowitz, "EMDR: Taking a Closer Look," *Scientific American*, December 6, 2007, 1, http://www.scientificamerican.com/article/emdr-taking-a-closer-look/.

14. Shari Roan ("The Thirty-Day Myth," *Los Angeles Times*, November 10, 2008) cites several studies, including Bennett Fletcher's 1999 research conducted for NIDA's Drug Abuse Treatment Outcome Studies, which showed that after ninety days in recovery centers, the relapse rate dropped steadily the longer a person was in treatment; and a 2001 study, conducted by UCLA of 1,167 adolescent substance users in rehabilitation centers, which showed that those who were in treatment for ninety days were subsequently less likely to relapse than those who were in rehab for only twenty-one days.

15. SAMHSA, "Affordable Care Act Update," *SAMHSA News* 22, no. 1 (Winter 2014), http://www.samhsa.gov/samhsaNewsLetter/Volume_22_Number_1/affordable-care-act-update.aspx#.VDmun5ZMFjA.

16. Peter Luongo, Executive Director of the Institute for Research, Education & Training in Addictions, quoted in Smith and DeMio, "No way out: Heroin addicts trapped in deadly maze," *Cincinnati Enquirer*, May 19, 2014.

Chapter Seven

· · · · · · · · ·

Gender-Specific Treatment: A Growing Trend

"With regard to treatment, few young adults will follow through with referrals if they feel the treatment modality (type) is irrelevant to their situation."[1] Several studies have shown gender-responsive programs to be more effective than mixed-gender facilities for women, and this is the case both in terms of retaining them and in equipping them for life after treatment.[2] Yet only about 38 percent of treatment facilities have targeted women-only programs. Crucially, there is a scarcity of programs for pregnant or post-partum women, particularly if they have other children, which is of course a barrier to many women substance-abusers.

I have previously discussed what practices are most effective in treatment centers and as therapies for addiction, as well as the fact that at this time there is not a standardized set of requirements for treatment centers. Instead, we have a vast menu of options, many of which have not implemented current evidence-based approaches. Now let's take a closer look at what we know about the specific needs of women.

Less than a century ago there was next to no help for anyone with a substance use disorder, let alone any recognition of the differences between genders as well as age groups. For roughly the first third of the twentieth century, addiction was an intractable medical problem and those who were addicted most often died of the disease. A few private psychiatric hospitals, rest homes, and sanitariums took in people of means, serving basically as glorified drying-out centers. In 1935, two men, Dr. Robert Smith and Bill Wilson, both of whom had a severe drinking problem, discovered they could quit drinking by talking honestly to each other about their cravings and reaching out to talk to other, still-sick alcoholics. This simple idea, like many revolutionary changes, grew into Alcoholics Anonymous, the first twelve-step fellowship, and later into its many sister programs (Narcotics Anonymous, Gamblers Anonymous, Overeaters Anonymous, etc.) that have given millions of people productive lives in recovery in more than 170 countries.

But where were the women? In reality women have always been part of the group of people suffering from substance abuse. In fact, women made up the majority of drug users in the late nineteenth century when opium and morphine, often in the form of laudanum, was dispensed by doctors and over-the-counter to treat "feminine hysteria"—painful menstrual periods, and the like. An estimated 300,000 women became addicted and many overdosed.[3] It was less stigmatizing for women in that era to use opium, morphine, or laudanum than it was to consume alcohol. Men could drink in public at bars; women who did so were not considered respectable. Yet many women did drink, behind closed doors. A handful of groups, notably the Martha Washington Societies—a social reform group formed in the 1840s by working-class women to aid poor families—took female drunkenness seriously, visiting homes to try to help wives and mothers achieve "temperance."

As a result of the vast changes in the twentieth century—including the Roaring Twenties and the greater independence of women during World War II—women came out of the shadows. They went to speakeasies, nightclubs, and dances; they drank cocktails and used drugs; some left home to go to college or find employment. But women alcoholics remained highly stigmatized and still tended to drink in secret. Even when twelve-step groups first appeared, female addicts—and their families—continued to try to hide the problem. Marty Mann, a pioneering woman member of Alcoholics Anonymous, said women alcoholics in the 1930s and 1940s cared "almost pathologically" about what others would think of them.[4] A gifted public speaker, Mann played a vital role in shaping American policy toward treating alcoholism as a disease—a revolutionary concept back then—and ending the double standard for women substance-abuse sufferers.

A few desperate and brave women did turn to twelve-step meetings. It was a huge step for them and a big step for the fellowship to accept women into the program. In their early days twelve-step groups would meet in members' homes and clubhouses, and wives would come along and gather in the kitchen, leading to the birth of Al-Anon. When a few women alcoholics showed up, nobody was sure what to do with them. Some of the wives complained that "loose women" would mingle with their husbands. At first, the female alcoholics stayed in the kitchen with the wives, but when the book *Alcoholics Anonymous* (affectionately called the "Big Book" by AA members) was published in 1939, a story of a female member's alcoholism and recovery was included among twenty others. The book unequivocally notes the faster pace of alcoholism in women: "Potential female alcoholics often turn into the real thing and are gone beyond recall in a few years."[5] The latest edition of the "Big Book" was published in 2001, and it includes a dozen stories by women who have entered recovery, including young women.

Still, much of the language of the book is based on a male perspective. Informally, some women twelve-step group members interpret the recovery literature in ways that are nurturing for them. There has been a growing understanding, with the help of addiction specialists such as Stephanie Covington and Brenda Iliff, that, generally speaking, women in recovery need validation rather than ego-deflation.[6] As an example, take the First Step of the twelve-step program Alcoholics Anonymous: "We admitted that we were powerless over alcohol—that our lives had become unmanageable" (Narcotics Anonymous substitutes "our addiction" for "alcohol"). Because women have felt a lack of power historically, the word "powerless" can be problematic. Stephanie Covington, a leader in the field of developing literature and therapeutic techniques that speak to women's needs, points out that this "powerlessness" needs to be carefully explained to female newcomers as referring specifically to having no control over substances and the resulting behavior. In admitting that, women will gain self-knowledge and self-worth, so that the First Step actually leads to a new kind of empowerment. A recent study supports Covington's thesis: Learning to cope with negative emotions turns out to be most important for women, whereas learning to deal with high-stress situations is more key for men.[7]

That legions of women have taken this approach to "working the program" is clear. Today, women make up between one third to one half of AA's membership worldwide, which is open to all races, ethnicities, faiths or non-faith, and sexual orientations.

Rehabilitation centers grew out of a response to the growth of the twelve-step recovery movement. In 1949, the venerable Hazelden Center first opened its doors to treat "curable alcoholics of the professional class"—in other words, white males. A few years later, in 1956, Hazelden opened a small women-only unit. Slowly, acceptance of the idea of addiction as a treatable disorder grew until, in the 1970s, federal legislation finally recognized alcoholism as a disease, and treatment facilities became widely available as a result.

Most if not all of these rehab or treatment centers founded their approach to recovery on the existing research, which was based on the experiences of male alcoholics, bolstered by the results of a 1946 survey called the "Jellinek Curve." The survey asked recovering alcoholics specific questions, including how their alcoholism had progressed and how it had been arrested. Crucially, a small percentage of the survey results were not used in the final report because they were deemed "too different"—too much at variance with the majority of responses. In time, a fresh look at these unused reports revealed they had all come from women respondents.[8] In the words of a recent landmark publication on women and addiction: "Historically, substance abuse was seen as a male problem, and as a result, treatment programs were and continue to be designed primarily for men and by men."[9]

It wasn't that many women weren't getting well in twelve-step programs. Thanks in part to its loose, tolerant format, the fellowships grew into programs where the "men stick with the men" and "the women stick with the women," which fostered a network of supportive and empathic fellow-travelers. When I got into recovery in the late 1970s in the "rooms" of the fellowship, the community of women, especially during my early, more vulnerable period, was crucial, and a wonderful gift given freely. It continues to be so for vast numbers of women as well as men. Twelve-step programs have validated and valued women's experiences and needs, and twelve-step fellowships often display a genuine openness to new voices and experiences (such as addiction to drugs other than alcohol). By the 1970s many women were emboldened to share their experiences with alcohol and drug use, and First Lady Betty Ford led the way when she broke the taboo and publicly announced she had been treated for alcoholism and prescription pill addiction. Betty Ford was determined to offer programs for women, as well as men, at the famous treatment center that bears her name. Its website echoes her thinking: "Key barriers that get in the way of a woman accessing care are: family, money, shame, denial. . . . They are all interrelated and important."[10]

Since then, and especially since the 1990s, a growing number of both medical and social scientists have studied the effects of drugs and alcohol on girls and women and how their needs can be met to recover. According to a leading publication, "Understanding how substance abuse affects women of all ages . . . is essential if we are successfully to improve the quality of life for millions of women and their families."[11]

And yet, the model in place in treatment facilities today is often still the male-based approach from an earlier generation—even in mixed-gender settings. As Stephanie Covington and others have described, women addicts tend to feel cloaked in shame, even self-abasement, whereas "men who are addicted typically build up grandiose false selves that must be challenged before they can discover and cultivate their true selves. . . . Many practitioners who have studied men often see [all] addicts as self-focused, and perceive their task as breaking that obsession with self."[12] But women are not necessarily well-served by such techniques.

We are learning more and more not only about the relevance of gender issues for female substance users, but for males as well. Some therapists are even challenging the traditional confrontational approach for men—particularly for young men. Talk therapies are a case in point. Gender-stereotyping behavior by adults leads many boys to hold back expressing emotions of pain, grief, or hurt. Furthermore, brain research suggests "the locus of brain activity associated with negative emotion remains stuck in the amygdala [the part of the brain that processes emotional reactions]. Asking a seventeen-year-old boy to explain why he's feeling glum may be as productive as asking a six-year-old boy the same question."[13]

Significantly, anger is one emotion young males are allowed to express, often cultivated through teen sports. Injury, homicide, and suicide rates are higher among males than females, though over their lifespan, women are three times more likely than men to attempt suicide. Boys in trouble with substance use—more than one in four young men between the ages of eighteen and twenty-five report dependence—could also benefit from non-traditional approaches to treatment in single-sex settings. Critics of the "old system" say what is needed is a safe, male-only environment that challenges belief systems about what it means to be male, teaching young men how to open up and create bonds with other men, as well as how to deal with anger. In addition, an all-male staff could break the cycle of men relying exclusively on women to meet their emotional needs. Caron Recovery is one example of a treatment center with a program for adult men (ages twenty-one and over) that aims not only to treat addiction, but also to teach emotional skills and ways to express feelings in a healthy way.[14]

"In our experience generally, young women are more treatment-ready than men," young-adult addiction therapist Tom Deitzler told me, adding they are also—and what parent of a daughter doesn't know this—more likely to talk. A young woman's developing brain differs from a young man's in a way that may make her more able to articulate her emotions in treatment. While negative emotions are, as it were, stuck in the young male's brain, in young women, more negative emotion is engaged in the cerebral cortex. In plain English, she's able to explain her sadness, while her male counterpart is not yet ready to. There is one significant caveat: When young women and men are in mixed-gender recovery groups, women tend to disengage and are less likely to discuss trauma and sexual abuse in the presence of men. Women are far likelier to talk about shame-filled events in their lives in an all-female setting. In practical terms, young women and men in early recovery may become focused on—or obsessed with—a member of the opposite sex instead of focusing on why they are in rehab—an added impediment, as it's hard enough to get a person in treatment to focus on themselves without distractions. (Note also that LGBT women benefit from counselors who understand their particular issues.)

My daughter's first experience in a treatment center bears out the pitfalls of mixed-gender rehabs at the most basic level. Even with living quarters at opposite ends of a large building, the boys and girls showed real creativity in circumventing the rules and finding ways to get together. In twelve-step culture there is an unofficial "thirteenth step" that refers to the time-honored dance of hormones: guys in the program hitting on "newbie" women and vice versa. With "women stick with the women" as an unofficial rule, women with some recovery under their belt help those new to the program avoid the pitfalls of sex and romance, since relationship problems in early recovery often lead to using again.

In same-gender recovery environments women find:

First: "An understanding of the differences in the ways in which girls develop their identities and self-concepts is critical when assessing or creating treatment plans."[15]

Second: "A program that focuses on the needs of a young adult of either gender may have better outcomes. When a program focuses on a woman's problems, she is more likely to complete treatment than women in mixed-gender programs."[16]

Sometimes a young woman will balk at going to a women-only recovery center or program. The roots of this resistance may be subconscious—she may not want to find out about herself. Common complaints are, "I don't want to be with *just* women," "I don't like women," and "Women are catty." But evidence is compelling that the biological, emotional, and social differences between the sexes make for a strong case for separate treatment for young women and men. Many will have suffered physical and sexual violence and may have contracted a sexually-transmitted disease or experienced an unplanned pregnancy. Their shame tends to lessen when they are with other women who share similar experiences.

Reassure a young woman balking at a women-only facility that she will not be living in a cloister. During the twenty-eight to ninety days she'll spend in active treatment, she'll be encouraged to attend "off-campus" mixed-gender meetings of twelve-step groups, where she can interact with young men in a supervised, safe structure to prepare her for the post-treatment time back in the "real world."

Diane, a twenty-five-year-old recovering alcohol and cocaine abuser, says: "I needed time to remember who I was without the drugs and alcohol. I think what helped the most was the other young women who were there with me. As a young woman in full-blown addiction, most of my time was spent either with men or with unhealthy women. Because my recovery center was run by women, I felt empowered and my self-esteem as a woman improved dramatically. The things I didn't want to face while I was in it ended up being necessary for me to grow and change."

As addiction specialist Tom Deitzler put it to me in one conversation, "Overall, women have experienced a deeper progression of their addiction and more trauma. And most young women need longer-term care." New findings in recent years about what is most effective in treating both genders are leading to the development of gender-specific programs by long-established recovery centers as well as new ones. These recovery centers can vary widely in their approaches, and it's worth repeating: No one therapeutic approach works for everyone.

Now let's take a closer look at some of the leading recovery centers with women-targeted programs.

A Closer Look at Four Women's Recovery Programs

While doing the research for this book and during my daughter's recovery, I took a closer look at several recovery centers with different approaches and good reputations. Following is an overview of four programs, all of which accept insurance and have varying degrees of scholarship help, with brief discussions of their different emphases and a summary of their unique features. As you read about these, keep in mind that even in the best environment, a young woman in treatment can flourish or fail to succeed for a host of reasons.

Orchid Recovery Center for Women

(Acquired in 2014 by Palm Partners Treatment Center, but retains its character.)

In Florida, there are, it seems, as many rehabilitation centers, halfway houses, and sober living facilities as there are sandy beaches (California has even more). Walking along the shore in Palm Beach or Delray Beach at sunset, chances are you'll come upon a group of young people sitting in a circle. This is likely to be a twelve-step meeting of some of the thousands of young adults new in recovery or with longer-term recovery who have attended rehab centers in Florida. Among them, the Orchid Recovery Center for Women is a pioneer in female-specific treatment of a range of addictions. It's a small, intimate place, treating just eighteen women at a time, a good proportion of them young adults aged eighteen and over. Founded in the 1990s by Julie Queler, herself a recovering addict, the Orchid program is based on the insights of epidemiologist and addiction specialist Dr. Karen Dodge.

Dr. Dodge was one of the first to address the lack of addiction research conducted specifically on women. During her doctoral research at Florida International University in the 1990s, she found a significant correlation between addiction and low self-esteem, depression and, most importantly, lack of a social support network for women. Inspired by Dr. Dodge's work, the Orchid developed a philosophy based on relational growth, with the guiding premise that addiction damages and even destroys the very support network a woman needs to be healthy. The goal is to help newly-recovering women learn to trust each other and build interdependence in ways that speak to the feminine experience.

A recently added component to the Orchid is Hormonal Awareness Therapy, based on emerging research about the debilitating, sometimes devastating, effects of hormonal changes on addicted and recovering women at different phases of the menstrual cycle—with a focus on helping newly-recovering women recognize their symptoms and find effective tools to cope without relapsing.

Coaching women in how to process trauma is also key to treatment at the Orchid, achieved through a mixture of cognitive behavioral therapy and healing arts, such as psychodrama, acupuncture, yoga and exercise, massage, conscious eating and nutrition, family sessions, and spiritual guidance. The aim is to allow women to safely and rapidly become aware of limiting and destructive patterns and learn to replace them with more rewarding thoughts and behavior.

Treatment at the Orchid is firmly grounded in the twelve-step recovery program. After women have been medically detoxed and monitored at a nearby detoxification center, they move to a cluster of small villas aptly called the "Bloom." Designed according to the Planetree Model (of healthcare facility design), the physical space is a deliberate part of the treatment in which beauty and calm are said to promote both the lessening of negative feelings and the process of healing by improving mood, immune system response, and cognition. Lush plantings and mellow tropical colors provide a soothing aesthetic environment not often seen at rehabilitation centers. Beds are draped with soft, airy netting, a pretty cocoon that also opens into the bedrooms, providing a nurturing place for women at this vulnerable time in their lives.

During the day, women attend the varied therapeutic offerings; travel together to supervised off-site twelve-step meetings, grocery stores, beaches, shopping centers, concerts, and picnics; learn to prepare healthy meals; have fun; and deepen their new friendships.

Good treatment centers stress the importance of continued care after the initial treatment of thirty to ninety days. Many of the women graduating from the Orchid move on to sober/recovery houses, which coordinate care with their counselors and offer continued therapy, relapse prevention workshops, and gradual, stepped-down supervision in the sharing of responsibilities, finding jobs, attending school, and interacting with peers.

www.orchidrecoverycenter.com
West Palm Beach, Florida

The Caron Center's Female Young Adult Program

The Caron Center in Wernersville, Pennsylvania, is one of the oldest established large treatment centers to treat young female and male populations separately. Caron began as "Chit Chat Farm" in 1959, when Richard Caron, a wealthy recovering alcoholic, and his wife bought a stately resort hotel in the rolling hills of Wernersville. By 2006, Caron opened a young adult female program for ages twenty to twenty-five, as well as a young adult male program in an attractive, clean setting. In addition, there are gender-separate (girls only/boys only) and gender-specific programs for ages thirteen to nineteen, with onsite, licensed, alternative education, and extended care if needed to treat addiction, co-occurring mental health issues, family conflict, low self-esteem, cutting, anger, and body image issues.

Today Caron provides treatment at facilities in Wernersville, Pennsylvania, Princeton, Texas, and Boca Raton, Florida. The Caron Renaissance Center in Boca Raton serves ages eighteen and over and includes an optional College Bound Program, in which individual education plans are designed for patients (at no extra charge), either during or after treatment.

Caron's Wernersville program includes an adolescent unit for ages thirteen to nineteen, which takes place in a separate facility. Its program for single women, ages twenty to twenty-five, without children who are dependent on their families is highly structured throughout the day. During periods of free time, patients must travel in groups of three. Along with the therapeutic plan offered in the Adult Women's program (for women ages twenty-six and older), the Young Adult program adds a life skills component and emphasizes the treatment of traumatic issues. "Our highest-rated life skill is exposing trauma. And a majority of the girls are traumatized," the program director, Tom Deitzler, told me.

Peer involvement is especially emphasized: "New patients are matched up with others further on in the program who used the same substances, who share their experience, strength, and hope, and help the newer patient not to isolate." According to director Deitzler, since the peer culture system was put in place the completion rate for the program increased. Along with attendance at twelve-step meetings, there are recreational activities such as going to the movies, bowling, working out at the gym, and going on overnight and adventure-based trips. "This population can feel lost about having fun after discharge," Deitzler said. Caron also has a program especially designed for relapsers.

For Caron, family participation for both the young adult female and the separate young adult male programs is mandatory, according to Deitzler: "The family member who is motivated for treatment for a daughter should call us. We give the family a pre-family screening, an admissions screening, and a bio-social assessment. Parents have to feel safe before their involvement in the treatment. The biggest fear is of family secrets being exposed, so parents are often mentored into treatment, beginning with pre-family program anxiety. We dance with the resistance. The thing we offer the family is hope, self-respect, and dignity to the family system. And we have better than 99 percent family participation. We have a Saturday and Sunday forum for education of the family: family structure work, a timeline of their daughter's use, and, after treatment, a complete analysis."

Extended care is offered at the Wernersville, Pennsylvania, and the Boca Raton, Florida, facilities.

www.caron.org
Wernersville, Pennsylvania (main campus)

The Hazelden Center's Women's Recovery Program, and The Center for Youth and Families

(In 2013 Hazelden and The Betty Ford Center merged to form The Hazelden Betty Ford Foundation, becoming the largest nonprofit addiction center in the country.)

Hazelden is located about fifty miles north of St. Paul, Minnesota, in Center City, with a large complex of institutional-looking buildings that serve about 2,000 substance abusers a year. In addition to its structured, group-oriented ethos, it offers a pool, fitness center, meditation room, café, store, and lounges.

In 2006, the same year that the Caron Center opened its Young Adult Female program, Hazelden opened an expanded Women's Recovery Center for women aged eighteen and over, with three twenty-two-bed units and a twenty-two-bed extended care unit. (Like the Caron Center, Hazelden has established centers elsewhere, including New York City.)

According to their website, "It has been Hazelden's experience, supported by subsequent and ongoing research, that gender-specific treatment provides patients with the best opportunity for recovery from alcohol and drug addiction." Though the genders mix at many meetings and activities, one of the rules is no talking to the opposite sex.

In terms of young people in general, Hazelden has been treating males and females aged fourteen to twenty-five since 1981 at the Center for Youth and Families. Set on the shores of Medicine Lake in Plymouth, Minnesota, the Center treats thirty males and fifteen females in separate twenty-eight-day programs, along with a suggested program for parents and siblings. According to the website, "Concerned by shifting patterns of teen drug abuse and a shortage of treatment options for young addicts, we have to do something."[17] An additional thirty-two-bed unit was recently built to serve young women at the Center for Youth and Families. Parents should note that depending on the initial and ongoing assessment of a young female patient, she might be placed in either the Women's Recovery Center in Center City or the Center for Youth and Families in Plymouth.

Reputable recovery facilities always address the impact of addiction on loved ones. In addition to optional programs for parents, Hazelden also offers one for siblings, where they can share with peers, as well as Teen Intervene, for young people who have engaged in mild to moderate chemical use and are not yet addicted. Teen Intervene comprises three ninety-minute, one-on-one sessions with a counselor, and parents are invited to participate in the final session. Hazelden also provides its clients with eighteen months of free support after treatment from a licensed addiction counselor, via the internet and telephone.

www.hazelden.org
Center City, Minnesota, main campus (adults)
Plymouth, Minnesota, main campus (youth)

The Hazelden Betty Ford Foundation

This famous recovery center in Rancho Mirage, California, opened in 1982, founded by First Lady Betty Ford after her own recovery and landmark public acknowledgement of her treatment. The Betty Ford Center treats a maximum of forty patients at any given time and features a young adult track for those aged eighteen to twenty-five in gender-separate areas.

Although the Center has attracted many of the rich and famous, including well-known actors, it is known for keeping to a strict schedule in a rather clinical setting, with a doctor on site and nurses present around the clock. The young adults get up at 6:30 a.m. for chores and breakfast, then attend a co-ed step meeting and daily topic lecture, followed by a variety of group therapy sessions, including special groups for eating disorders, trauma, grief, self-esteem, and other topics, as well as offerings of biofeedback, meditation, acupuncture, gym, yoga, and fitness. The day wraps up at 9:00 p.m. Notably, the Center mandates longer treatment for young adult women than for young men. The website explains that young adult women stay in inpatient care twice as long as men—sixty days as opposed to thirty—because experience has shown women need longer care to heal from trauma and loss. After taking part in a trauma and addiction workshop, they transition to aftercare at a residential day treatment. At this point in their early recovery, patients plan outings, and many continue on a specialized treatment track.

There is also a Family Program for family members aged thirteen and older, consisting of five days of intensive meetings, Monday through Friday, and a program for younger children in the family, ages seven to twelve. As an incentive to participate, the cost of a family member for the Family Program is included in each patient's cost of treatment.

www.bettyfordcenter.org
Rancho Mirage, California

Takeaways

The Orchid Recovery Center: Women-only, eighteen and older. Very gender-responsive. Stresses "relational group" treatment modalities designed for women and holistic treatment, including Hormonal Awareness Therapy.

The Caron Center: Separates by age: thirteen to nineteen, twenty to twenty-five, and twenty-six and older. Some gender-specific treatment. Stresses life skills, including trauma healing for young women, peer involvement, and mandatory family participation for young adults aged twenty to twenty-five.

The Hazelden Women's Recovery Center: For ages eighteen and older. There is a women's unit at a separate Center for Youth and Families with gender-specific counseling. The Center provides eighteen months of free post-program support from an addiction counselor via telephone and internet.

The Hazelden Betty Ford Foundation: The youth program is for eighteen- to twenty-five-year-olds, with gender-separate living quarters. Thirty days for males, sixty days for females, including a trauma and addiction workshop.

Notes on Chapter Seven

1. Cynthia A. Briggs, and Jennifer L. Pepperell, *Women, Girls, and Addiction: Celebrating the Feminine in Counseling Treatment and Recovery* (New York and London: Routledge, 2009), 119.

2. C. E. Grella, "Women in Residential Drug treatment," *Journal of Health Care for the Poor and Underserved* 10, no. 2 (1999): 216–29, as quoted in www.caron.org/sites/caron.orgfiles/womenaddiction on a comparison of 4,000 women in gender-separate and mixed-gender treatment programs.

3. Andrew Kolodny, MD, Chief Medical Officer of Phoenix House Academy, and President of Physicians for Responsible Opioid Prescribing (PROP), in a talk at Phoenix House Academy, March 15, 2014.

4. Sally Brown and David R. Brown, *The First Lady of Alcoholics Anonymous* (Center City, MN: Hazelden, 2001), 100.

5. *Alcoholics Anonymous*, 4th ed. (Alcoholics Anonymous World Services, Inc., 2001), 33.

6. See Stephanie S. Covington, *A Woman's Way through The Twelve Steps* (Center City, MN: Hazelden, 1994), and Brenda Iliff, *A Woman's Guide to Recovery* (Center City, MN: Hazelden, 2008).

7. John F. Kelly and Bettina B. Hoeppner, "Does Alcoholics Anonymous work differently for men and women? A moderated multiple-mediation analysis in a large clinical sample," *Drug and Alcohol Dependence* 130 (June 1, 2013): 186–93.

8. MARR Recovery Center's Website, "Women and Addiction: Surrounded by Shame," May 24, 2012, www.marrinc.org/women-and-addiction.

9. National Center on Addiction and Substance Abuse at Columbia University (CASA), *Women Under the Influence* (Baltimore, MD: Johns Hopkins University Press, 2005), 132.

10. The Betty Ford Center's Website, "Women: Overcoming Barriers To Treatment," December 1, 2009, http://www.bettyfordcenter.org/recovery/treatment/women-overcoming-barriers-to-treatment.php.

11. CASA, *Women under the Influence*, 2005.

12. Stephanie S. Covington, "Helping Women Recover: Creating Gender-Responsive Treatment," in *The Handbook of Addiction Treatment for Women: Theory and Practice*, S. L. A. Straussner and S. Brown (eds.) (San Francisco: Jossey-Bass, 2002), 4. Reprinted with permission.

13. Leonard Sax, *Why Gender Matters: What Parents and Teachers Need to Know about the Emerging Science of Sex Differences* (New York: Doubleday, 2005), 29.

14. See OneCircleFoundation.org for more on issues relevant to young men. See also Stephanie S. Covington, Dan Griffin, and Rick Dauer, *Helping Men Recover: A Program for Treating Addiction* (San Francisco: Wiley & Sons, 2011).

15. Briggs and Pepperell, *Women, Girls, and Addiction*, 137.

16. Ronald E. Claus, et al., "Does Gender-Specific Substance Abuse Treatment for Women Promote Continuity of Care?" *Journal of Substance Abuse Treatment* 32, no. 1 (January 2007): 27.

17. Jeremy Olson, "Hazelden Planning $30 Million Expansion at its Center for Teens," *Minneapolis Star Tribune*, September 6, 2011.

Chapter Eight

Special Considerations

Younger Girls, Ages Twelve to Seventeen

Almost three million of our youngest teens, ages twelve to seventeen, are addicted to alcohol or drugs. What puts them at particular risk? A recent study showed "the very plasticity of the adolescent brain that allows rapid learning and absorption of information also makes the brain vulnerable to outside stressors such as alcohol or drugs. . . . It takes more of a substance to get a high feeling when used by an adolescent . . . and there is a greater likelihood for the development of abuse or dependence."[1]

In this vulnerable population, prescription drugs including opioids, are found in family medicine cabinets or obtained from friends, dealers, physicians, or online pharmacies. Law enforcement officials lament the percentage of doctors who over-prescribe, a number of them criminally, and the easy availability of pills from unscrupulous online sources. (Legitimate online pharmacies can be found on a Drug Enforcement Agency (DEA) registered list.) The Federal government reports "nonmedical use of prescription and over-the-counter medicines remains a significant part of the teen drug problem. In 2013, 15 percent of high school seniors used a prescription drug non-medically."[2] As for marijuana, researchers speculate the active ingredient in the drug may interfere with the developing adolescent brain. Research found kids who smoked pot heavily (about four or more times per week) from the age of thirteen onward lost an average of eight IQ points.[3]

As mentioned earlier, teenage girls are at particular risk of addiction to painkillers: another study of three thousand teens in 2011 and 2012 found they were nearly twice as likely as boys to have misused them in the past year."[4] For girls, the current average age to start drinking, doing drugs, and developing eating disorders is about fifteen. It is no coincidence that "depression rates triple between ages of twelve and fifteen among adolescent girls," says a major new report, adding that an annual average of 1.4 million girls aged twelve to seventeen are three times more likely than boys their age to have experienced a major depressive episode in the past year (12 percent compared to 4.5 percent).[5] But despite the fact that the rate of both girls and boys seeking treatment has been steadily increasing since the mid-1990s, only two-fifths of girls aged fifteen to seventeen with depression and/or drug use received treatment, and only one-third of girls aged twelve to fourteen.

Many young addicted teenagers who do not get help—an estimated 36 percent—are simply not ready to stop using. The remainder either don't have any, or inadequate, health insurance, or are too ashamed to face the need for treatment. When they do enter treatment, girls are likelier to do so on their own or through their parents, while boys come to treatment more often through referrals by the criminal justice system.

Girls from about the age of twelve to seventeen need specific therapeutic approaches by recovery centers experienced in dealing with this age group's needs (such as body image disorders, cutting, bulimia, etc.). And there should be an accredited educational component for them to continue their schooling.

Studies have found both young girls and boys generally require a longer time in treatment than adults. Since normal adolescent physical, mental, and emotional development is delayed by mind- and mood-altering drugs, they frequently need help in developing life skills—how to develop concrete thinking and coping mechanisms, become responsible, and, not least, how to achieve healthy interpersonal relationships.

As we know, young women often need treatment for both depression and substance use disorder. However, because a young person's brain is still developing until about the age of twenty-four, she must be medicated under the careful supervision of a doctor who understands the medical aspects of addiction. Even "legitimate" drugs can be problematical for young people. Treatment with antidepressants and other medications can carry risks. As neuroscientist Dr. Amiz Raz cautions, "The human brain is developing exponentially when we are very young. And exposure to antidepressants may affect or influence the wiring of the brain, especially when it comes to certain elements that have to do with stress, emotion, and the regulation of these."[6] The Food and Drug Administration now requires such medication to carry a warning label about the risk of suicide for children and young adults aged eighteen to twenty-four.

High School and College Recovery Programs: A New Trend

"For teenagers," write researchers, "school often sits at the heart of the relapse threat."[7] True, so bitterly true, in my family's experience and for others I've known with addicted teenagers. In an attempt to deal with the sad reality that our kids may be offered drugs on their first day back at school post-rehab, "recovery schools" have been added in some school districts—there are currently some thirty addiction recovery high schools and less than twenty colleges nationally. The Association of Recovery Schools lists high schools and colleges that host such programs for young people after treatment at www.recoveryschools.org.

Recovery schools are commonly embedded within an existing school or set up as alternative school programs and provide an environment of peer support and ready access to counseling in addition to academics. Some are operated by recovery centers, such as the Phoenix House Academy of Westchester (New York), a residential high school that provides gender-specific services to some 160 drug-dependent boys and girls, ages fourteen to twenty. Parents of teenagers who are at-risk are encouraged to look within their own school districts and advocate for their child if need be. I mentioned my daughter attended a senior year alternative high school program for at-risk, underachieving bright students. Many of the students, but not all, were using drugs, and the hands-on, innovative, and caring attention of the teachers kept her and her friends engaged instead of possibly dropping out.

When a student returns to high school after treatment, parents should meet with the administration to plan the transition back to school and beyond. Be aware that several Federal laws exist to ensure services and to protect the privacy of a student during her re-entry: FERPA (Family Education Rights to Privacy Act) concerns the privacy of student education records; IDEA (Individuals with Disabilities Education Act) is designed to protect the rights of students with disabilities; and Section 504 of the Rehabilitation Act protects qualified individuals from discrimination based on their disability—including alcoholism and drug abuse.

The trend to build recovery schools is growing, along with a similar trend at the college level. "As many as one million college students nationwide meet the criteria for alcohol dependency and/or drug abuse," cites one researcher.[8] Binge drinking is a significant health issue among the college-age population in both genders. According to the Centers for Disease Control and Prevention, 11,500 people die every year as a result of binge drinking.

For college students in recovery, look for "sober" residences, meaning alcohol and drug-free floors in dorms and housing wherever possible. Texas Tech University's Center for the Study of Addiction and Recovery is considered the gold standard of comprehensive recovery programs for students aged eighteen to twenty-four. Texas Tech works with other colleges to implement their own recovery centers. The website of the Association of Recovery in Higher Education (CollegiateRecovery.org) lists the growing number of programs in place for students in recovery. Although still small, this is a growing trend in higher education. A recent example in New York City is the "Tribeca Twelve" (as in the Twelve Steps), a collegiate recovery residence for ages eighteen to twenty-nine operated by the Hazelden Center.

Young and Pregnant Women Substance Users

For all women of childbearing age, 5 percent were reported to have used illicit drugs in 2011. But in the fifteen- to seventeen-year-old group the rate was 20.9 percent, and in the eighteen to twenty-five age group, 8.2 percent.[9] Commenting on the frightening statistic of pregnant women who abuse opiates, one researcher exclaims, "The incidence has gone crazy. . . . People who previously might not have used heroin or the needle are more likely to use prescription opiates."[10] Pregnant women substance users face not only the risks of fetal alcohol syndrome, obstetric complications, and spontaneous abortion, but also arrest in some states, if they seek treatment and are found using substances, with the possibility of having their baby removed from their care and perhaps their other children as well. (In 2014, the governor of Tennessee signed a bill that could charge women with assault if they abuse narcotics while pregnant and give birth to a child who is drug-dependent or harmed. The bill was opposed by health organizations and women's rights advocates.) Because of this, women are urged to take methadone, the only treatment approved by the FDA for opioid dependency during pregnancy since 1995, although recently "buprenorphine [Suboxone] has been shown to result in fewer cases of NAS [physical dependence often resulting in Neonatal Abstinence Syndrome during the first week of life]."[11]

"Few doctors are willing to treat pregnant opiate addicts and there is no universally accepted standard of care for the babies."[12] However, a growing number of clinics in some states are treating pregnant women who are addicted. These clinics are often associated with university medical centers and are free for patients. Most pregnant women on heroin are put on methadone, while Suboxone is being used experimentally with others. Doctors, neonatal nurses, and treatment providers for this population point out that supporting the recovery of drug-addicted mothers is not just humane, but cost-effective, reducing the enormous expenses of health services, education, and many other social costs. In the absence of such much-needed post-natal care, family support is crucial.

Young Women Addicts with Children

Motherhood can pose a great challenge to a woman's treatment options. Historically, mothers who are alcoholics or drug addicts have been stigmatized, viewed as bad parents, and often unsupported—including by many professionals. Children can represent a barrier to treatment, since there may be no one to take care of them if the mother leaves to treat her illness. Also, many mothers are poor, with limited transportation and healthcare resources. See the Appendix for a list of resources that may be helpful.

Doreen's Story

Statistics indicate about one birth per hour is by young women with substance use disorder.[13]

Doreen is a twenty-six-year-old mother of a baby with serious health issues, and she is on methadone. Doreen's parents separated when she was about two years old and later divorced. Her father, Dan, a skilled craftsman, has always remained closely involved with Doreen. "My ex-wife was troubled. Her mother died when she was a teenager, and her father was a raging alcoholic." Dan made a point to see Doreen regularly when she was growing up, but she lived with her mother. "As I wasn't around full-time for Doreen's childhood—I was with her every weekend and other times—it's a grey area to me, but I knew my ex-wife had a pill problem, with Oxycontin and other pills. I would hear things about her being out of it, and she exhibited symptoms of a mood disorder, which I would learn about later. The ex-wife had no boundaries and didn't mature in a lot of ways; her family life had been shattered in one night. I found out my daughter started cutting herself at thirteen, as a freshman in high school." It was then that Dan got full custody of Doreen. "She went to a therapist, but I don't know how much good that did." When Doreen was a young woman, her mother died of an overdose. Meanwhile, Dan remarried and his current wife Karen has known Doreen from the time she was about ten. "Karen felt that Doreen, from the time she was a teenager, had a borderline personality. Later, I heard an expert speak about the disorder. She warned that these patients will chew up a therapist not trained to deal with it and she advocated inpatient treatment for the disorder and outpatient afterward." But Doreen was unwilling to do this.

"In high school, Doreen was smoking pot and using pills. She was not a drinker. I just figured she was going through that stage of life. There's some guilt I have about this. Then, she developed her own problem with Oxycontin, on and off, but she went to college and she went to a rehab. To my knowledge, she joined a twelve-step group in her early twenties, but I don't think she did the Steps. But to my knowledge, she had quit using. She had come back home and met a guy who was working and stable. He was laid-back, and she's a hurricane.

"Doreen was with this guy for several years, until about two and a half years ago. They'd set a date to get married in six months. She was working and had her own apartment; she had her ducks in a row. Then I remember one night we were at home, and she told me she had cold feet about getting married. She was full of doubts. And she said there was this other guy who she was involved with, who I didn't know about. And I didn't know he was a heroin addict. I wanted her to stay and talk about this, but she left to be with the new guy. Then, about a month later, while with Doreen and her stepmother, I get this call that she is using heroin. I was shocked. I couldn't believe this was going on.

"This thing caught me as a very big surprise. It was such a shock. And you think you can fix it. I was paying her debts, her car payments, giving her money. When she got evicted from her apartment, I went over there— if I hadn't gone all her stuff would have been thrown in the garbage. You get that bizarre thinking that you can fix it. She'd go in and out of detox, and I would take all of her clothes from her car, and have them all washed, and I'd clean the car. I was thinking I was putting the train back on the tracks. Externally, I was cleaning up all her messes. I look back now and see that I'd been enabling. I realize I was trying to alleviate my own fears, so I could sleep, so Doreen wouldn't go to jail for some of the things she had done with checks. And that turned out to be part of my enabling her. She was arrested a couple of times. She OD'd three times. Once I found out she shot up in the ER after she was taken in for an overdose! She went to a local rehab and calmed down after that. I thought.

"I started going to a twelve-step support group. A lot of people go to those thinking it's because of their kid's addiction, but it's for their own healing. The fellowship literature is extremely helpful. The group I go to is about twenty or so people, all dealing with the same thing. And there you meet all kinds of parents, solid nuclear families where one kid is doing well and the other is an addict. Good, wholesome parents. You never know. And then you look back and realize a lot of things you did were not helping. I was trading one mess to avoid another. If I had found the fellowship a lot earlier, I wouldn't have done a lot of things. Doreen tried to pit her stepmother against me. But it was clear to us that my daughter was in the wrong. Her stepmother is very stable, easy to talk to.

"I was open to doing anything that would help Doreen. We looked into rehabs, and she went to one that is well-known. But it didn't go too well. I couldn't visit due to a business obligation, but Karen was able to stay there for a day or two. The rehab called us up about doing the family component and about Doreen getting involved in an aftercare program. We were hoping when it came to the end at the rehab, Doreen would get set up in a sober house, or something like that. She'd told my wife she was really considering staying on so I was under that impression. But somebody sent her money, so the day she gets out of rehab, she has her plane ticket and everything set up, and she's right back to drugs. At the rehab we got a scholarship discount, but many people have told me, wow, you've just wasted a tremendous amount of money. At first, I looked at it that way. But later on I thought she might have died during that month of December if she had not gone to rehab.

"She got arrested again, and this time I was hoping she'd go to jail. As much as I was uncomfortable with that, it was either jail or the drugs. That day, she called me fifty times for bail. Fifty times! I never answered. I thought that little bit in jail might have an effect on her. But they released her after a day and a half. And she was back to living with the guy.

"The more Doreen used, the more I realized I had no control. She became part of a 'heroin couple.' Then she hit a crossroads, when she became pregnant two and a half years ago and decided she wanted to have the baby. The best thing that has happened to her was having a baby. She wasn't in a good place; she was on heroin. But she had to make a decision to stop using and get on a methadone maintenance program. So she did that. The baby has had serious health issues, but many of them have been resolved.

"Doreen has been good about all the hospital stuff and taking care of him, which is hard. She got into a program that provides transitional housing for women and children in need, where she pays a nominal rent. She advocates well for the baby, but she still exhibits immaturities. Some of her issues have never been resolved. I help her as I can.

"I would tell parents to go to a twelve-step meeting, hear from all the other parents that are experiencing the same thing, because a lot of people are at all different stages of where they're going with their child. You get to hear what they did in the beginning—the mistakes I felt I made in the beginning. It's almost like you can't help yourself, but then there comes a point where you just bite the bullet and don't feed the monster anymore. The literature is very insightful. And having a meditational program to deal with the stress has helped me immeasurably."

Ethnic and Multicultural Needs

In our heterogeneous society, cultural differences can impact all areas of medical treatment. Addiction treatment is no different. Treatment approaches need to be sensitive to race and culture.

For some immigrant women, language and culture is often a barrier. For Hispanic/Latina and Asian women, the value of family is greater than that of the individual. Culturally, motherhood is an exalted role, and giving up that role temporarily while in treatment, or losing custody, is especially stigmatizing. Therefore, strong support for family reunification is needed. African-American women face the impact of discrimination and obstacles such as the myth of the super-strong black woman in attaining recovery. This was the experience described by Chaney Allen in *I'm Black and I'm Sober*, where she tells the story of one woman's battle with discrimination and the obstacles of poverty in seeking and achieving recovery. Counselors advise that African-American women need "a gender-responsive, strengths-based model to develop or enhance a sense of empowerment by recognizing their assets and history of fortitude."[14]

Native American and Alaskan Native women suffer the highest rate of binge drinking, and drug use is also a serious problem. Those who are conversant with these cultures advise that treatment programs must treat both the individual and the culture and incorporate traditional spiritual practices such as sweat lodges and dancing, to be effective.[15]

Sexual Minorities

Jennifer Storm, a gay woman in recovery and author of *Blackout Girl: Growing Up and Drying Out in America* and *Leave the Light On: A Memoir of Recovery and Self-Discovery*, reports that many gay women use alcohol and other drugs to cover up painful feelings related to how society views members of the gay community and, in turn, how they view themselves.

"The culture of drinking and drugging within the LGBT community is a silent epidemic slowly killing many of its members."[16]

There are a few recovery centers that treat lesbian and bisexual women specifically. One is the Stonewall Institute in Phoenix, Arizona, which has an outpatient program especially for the LGBT community. Other resources are listed in the Appendix. For young women in general, "sexual orientation/identity should not be ignored in treatment and counselors should never assume that clients are heterosexual."[17]

Finding the appropriate kind of treatment for a teenaged or young adult daughter is paramount. A gender-separate facility is a good start, but, to be effective, the particular concerns of young women need to be addressed in a manner that "speaks" to them, and diagnosis and treatment are the frequently underlying issues. To be effective, the treatment plan should be individualized rather than "one size fits all," and a long-term plan should be developed. Relapse is common for young people in early recovery. In the next chapter we'll discuss some strategies to mitigate the potential for relapse, as well as to plan and prepare for its possibility.

Notes on Chapter Eight

1. Cynthia Briggs and Jennifer Pepperell, *Women, Girls, and Addiction: Celebrating the Feminine in Counseling Treatment and Recovery* (New York: Routledge, 2009), 48.

2. National Institute on Drug Abuse (NIDA), "Drug Facts: High School and Youth Trends," January 2014, http://www.drugabuse.gov/sites/default/files/drugfactsmtf.pdf.

3. "Troubling News for Young Stoners," *The Week*, September 14, 2012. Refers to a 2012 Duke University study of 1,000 people of various ages in New Zealand.

4. Mary Elizabeth Dallas, "Most Teens Who Misuse Painkillers Aren't After a High, Study Finds" *Health Day News*, November 13, 2013, http://consumer.healthday.com/kids-health-information-23/adolescents-and-teen-health-news-719/most-teens-who-misuse-pain-killers-aren-t-looking-for-a-high-study-finds-681966.html.

5. Substance Abuse and Mental Health Services Administration (SAMHSA), News Release, July 24, 2012. SAMHSA is in the process of preparing a comprehensive array of services to meet the needs of both young girls and boys, via the Child Mental Health Initiatives.

6. Quoted in Paul Raeburn, "Kids on Meds: Trouble Ahead," *Scientific American Mind* (June 2007), http://www.paulraeburn.com/articles/kids-on-meds-trouble-ahead/.

7. D. Paul Moberg and Andrew J. Finch, "Recovery High Schools: A Descriptive Study of School Programs and Students," *Journal of Groups in Addiction & Recovery*, 2 (2008): 128–61, http://www.ncbi.nlm.nih.gov/pmc/articles/PMC2629137.

8. David Unze, "St. Cloud State University Considers Recovery House," *St. Cloud Times*, February 13, 2011.

9. Denise J. Maguire, "Mothers on Methadone: Care in the NICU," *Neonatal Network* 32, no. 6, (November/December 2013): 409–15.

10. Marie J. Hayes, neuroscientist at the University of Maine, quoted in Pam Belluck's "Abuse of Opiates Soars in Pregnant Women," *The New York Times*, April 30, 2012.

11. Maguire, "Mothers on Methadone."

12. Abby Goodnough, "Newly Born and Withdrawing from Painkillers," *The New York Times*, April 9, 2011.

13. Stephen W. Patrick, et. al., "Neonatal Abstinence Syndrome and Associated Health Care Expenditures United States, 2000–2009," *Journal of the American Medical Association* 307, no. 18 (2012): 1934, doi:10.1001/jama.2012.3951.

14. SAMHSA, Center for Substance Abuse Treatment (CSAT), "Substance Abuse Among Specific Population Groups and Settings," in *Substance Abuse Treatment: Addressing the Specific Needs of Women. A Treatment Improvement Protocol (TIP)*, Report 51, revised edition (Rockville, MD: SAMHSA, 2012), 111. This report is a rich resource for many ethnicities.

15. As discussed in Teresa Milbrodt, "Breaking the Cycle of Alcohol Problems among Native Americans," *Alcoholism Treatment Quarterly* 20, no. 1 (2002): 19–32.

16. Victoria Brownworth, "Lesbians and Substance Abuse," *Curve* Magazine, 2010.

17. Thomas W. Irwin, "Sexual-Minority Women," in *Women and Addiction: A Comprehensive Handbook* edited by Kathleen T. Brady, Sudie E. Back, and Shelly F. Greenfield (New York: The Guilford Press, 2009), 486. Reprinted with permission.

Chapter Nine

· · · · · · · ·

Her Recovery Is a Dance,
Not a Straight Line

After my daughter completed treatment at her second inpatient treatment center, she moved into a sober house with other women new to recovery for several months. Then she began to chafe. Kim wanted her "freedom" and found a job and a small apartment and continued seeing her addiction counselor, even though the counselor and the house manager urged her to stay longer in her structured living arrangement. I agreed with their point of view, but she was determined to get out into the "real world." Another young woman, Sandy, age twenty-two, a recovering Oxycontin addict, points out that "keeping everyone in a safe little bubble in rehab keeps drugs and alcohol out, but it also keeps bad energy in. Women need to learn how to enter recovery in the real world."

New recovery can be complicated. Old-timers in twelve-step groups call this re-entry time the "pink cloud" syndrome, where the exhilaration of living drug and alcohol-free can tempt the newcomer into feeling cured. "My life filled out beautifully with new friends and fun, and gradually it got harder to take care of the basics like going to my support meetings," Kim admits. It took about a year, but eventually my daughter drifted away from recovery and back into drugs for a while, starting and stopping. Her experience is not unusual for young people and statistics reveal that most substance users who quit using will pick up again, though many of them will achieve recovery eventually. Treatment is not a cure. *There is no cure.* Had I known what I know today about the statistics for young women, I would have pressed harder for Kim to stay in a structured environment longer.

How to Increase the Odds of Her Long-term Success

The good news is that long-term treatment at a reputable rehab facility does translate into greater likelihood of staying in recovery. A UCLA study of adolescents treated for substance use disorder found those who were in treatment for ninety days or more had significantly lower relapse rates than those in programs of only twenty-one days.[1]

Practically speaking, young adult women benefit from enriched post-rehabilitation step-down programs and/or sober living situations where they learn life and coping skills and are called to be responsible for chores, finding employment or going to school, and continuing their aftercare, usually therapy and twelve-step meeting attendance. "For me, taking the step of going to a sober/halfway house was really important," says Sandy. "My ego was telling me I could take on the world, but in reality, the work starts once you leave rehab. Learning to live with other people was challenging, to say the least."

A young adult woman benefits in particular from learning new ways of thinking about situations (cognitive) and responding to them (behavioral). Painful feelings usually surface in recovery, ones that were blocked or numbed by self-destructive behavior and/or substance use in the past. An addictive personality is often tempted to cause chaos or excitement again—in part to divert herself from her feelings. Any of these factors can lead to picking back up. Learning not to act on impulse is key.

Relapse Prevention Programs

Relapse prevention programs are designed—both at outpatient and inpatient facilities—to help participants replace negative responses with positive ones. They teach proactive tools, including relaxation techniques like meditation, breathing exercises, yoga, and physical activity, as well as healthy eating habits. They also help recovering substance users learn to identify what "triggers" can move them toward wanting to use.

Stressors especially dangerous for women include interpersonal losses, such as a death, separation, romantic problems, and peer pressure. Stressors especially dangerous for men are feeling "too" good during "happy connecting" occasions. Stressors common to women and men are being hungry, tired, feeling angry, lonely or bored, starting a job, being criticized, and having an argument. I personally remember feeling as if my nerves were outside my skin in early recovery. Minor slights and remarks could set me off, and several times I came close to drinking over incidents that I can't even recall today.

"Stressors" or "triggers" for a woman new to recovery can be physical, mental or emotional—in other words, the whole person is affected by the illness of addiction. Therefore, healing and recovery need to be holistic and take into account the differences between the genders. For example, since peer relationships are so important for female teens and young adult women, having a network of fellow women friends in recovery can make all the difference for her.

Sober/Recovery Living Houses

My daughter lived in a sober/recovery house after her second inpatient treatment. For both women and men fresh out of treatment, living with other recovering individuals of the same gender in a highly structured, family-style environment with supervised activities can be a great benefit. Many sober living houses or transitional living houses are privately owned in residential areas, offering private or shared rooms at affordable rates. (Note that while the terms "sober/recovery house" and "halfway house" are often used interchangeably, there are differences. A halfway house is technically financed by behavioral health insurance, while a sober house is not billable to health insurance.) The house she chooses should have firm rules and clear consequences for breaking them. There should be zero tolerance for drug and alcohol use (with random drug and alcohol testing), for violence, theft, sex on the premises, for curfew violation, and for unexcused absences. Household tasks are shared and personal responsibility is stressed, along with peer group recovery support. Unless there is a compelling reason, a resident should be required to work, or to be actively looking for work, or be a student and must attend a minimum number of weekly peer-support and house meetings.

If this is an option you want to pursue for your daughter, get involved. In my experience and those of other parents I've talked to, a sober house is only as good as the people running it, and the amount of practical real-life help it can offer. First, look for a house that is monitored, either by the recovery center that refers its clients there, or by sober living coalitions that maintain peer reviews and inspections. Second, make sure the residence is clean and orderly, with onsite recovery management. I am always uneasy when I hear of young people in recovery for less than five years living together in a "sober house." It takes tough angels with a lot of time and energy to help "newbies" manage the roller-coaster of early recovery.

Of the estimated 45,000 to 60,000 beds in sober houses nationwide, less than 20 percent are designated for women and even fewer are specifically geared toward mothers with children. Nevertheless, a mixed-gender sober house is not a good idea for young women, for the same reasons it's not a good idea for them to be in a mixed-gender rehab.

I was encouraged by my visit to Kim's sober house in southern Florida during her free time. I found a tidy, spotless, rather modest home with a comfortable living room and well-ordered kitchen and dining space and a large yard. My daughter's shared bedroom was neat as a pin (unimaginable to me after the chaos that was her room at home when she was using). There were daily house meetings and required twelve-step recovery meetings, as well as scheduled trips to doctors and therapists. In hindsight, I could have interacted more with the manager of the house who, to her everlasting credit, strived to keep in constant contact with her ten to twelve charges. I did not want to intrude too much on the proceedings, or on my daughter's newborn recovery. As a result I missed the opportunity to ask some important questions. For example, how did the management of the house help these women new to recovery find jobs? The residents (as is the case in most sober living arrangements) had to leave the house from 9:00 a.m. to 5:00 p.m. and "look for work" or apply to a nearby community college or find volunteer work. They had to call in to the house manager, but that was the extent of the supervision. My daughter later confessed she and others sometimes spent their time "hanging out" at the beach.

My greatest concern was about what would happen to women who broke the cardinal rule and were found to have used a substance. You hear about so many kids who relapse (or "slip") once, and then they're kicked out of a program. This seems tragically counterintuitive to me because relapse is a predictable occurrence in dealing with addiction; therefore, it should be planned for by the recovery center and/or sober house. Folks who relapse and have to leave their support center are often placed in a detox or another recovery center or a hospital. Sometimes they are shipped home. But often, tragically, they end up on the streets. Since this is the sad reality of the kind of treatment that is available, parents have to anticipate this possibility and have a plan in place in the event it happens. I encourage parents to ask pointed questions of the facilities where their children will be housed while entering recovery.

Recovery Support: Twelve-Step and Other Mutual Support Recovery Groups

All mutual support programs are free, are located all over the country, and are comprised of people who tend to share the same focus: to stay in recovery and build a healthy life. In twelve-step programs a "sponsor" is another recovering individual of the same gender with more recovery time under her belt who can help guide the "sponsee" through the program of recovery based on the Twelve Steps and encourage her to build a support network of like-minded friends in the fellowship. A sponsor is not intended to be a therapist, medical expert, substitute parent, or even a friend, although many close friendships grow from the relationship.

Most twelve-step groups are mixed-gender, but there are often men's and women's only meetings; young people's groups; and LGBT meetings (among others). There is a dynamic organization called the International Conference of Young People in Alcoholics Anonymous (ICYPAA.org) that promotes recovery and fellowship among its members with dances, conventions, and more. Encourage your child to attend a variety of meetings in order to find the one that suits her best and that she is most comfortable with.

Other groups that promote recovery include
- Secular Organizations for Sobriety (SOS) (SOSSobriety.org);
- Rational Recovery (Rational.org), which offers courses via its website;
- Self-Management and Recovery Training (SMART) (SmartRecovery.org); and
- Women for Sobriety (WFS) (WomenForSobriety.org), who address the special needs, struggles, and issues of women in recovery. Unfortunately, there are not many WFS groups around.

Peer Recovery Support Coaching is a concept where both volunteers and paid peer leaders in recovery offer social support services to a peer who is new in recovery. The Substance Abuse and Mental Health Services Administration (SAMHSA) funds grant projects around the country to develop and deliver such services through the Recovery Community Services Program (RCSP). While a twelve-step sponsor guides the newly recovering person through the steps of a recovery program, a peer leader is there to offer practical support and guidance, but not directives or therapy. In 2014, a national accreditation council began awarding organizations that meet its standards.[2] This is in recognition of the fact that so many adults, and young adults, need help in almost every area of their lives to strengthen fledgling recovery and become productive. A peer support leader can help with finding sober housing, improving job skills, enrolling in educational programs, making new friends, organizing free time, and budgeting—in short, all of the life skills that can be daunting and yet are so important for a young woman in recovery. Check with her county, city or state for the Recovery Community Services Program offerings in her area. Some states currently require insurance plans to reimburse clients who use these services.

Counseling/Therapy

Counseling, either individual or group, with a psychotherapist, psychiatrist, social worker, or other counselor who is trained in addiction is a useful tool for women new in recovery. For those who have other issues in addition to addiction—such as depression, anxiety, eating disorders, bipolar disorder, or other challenges—therapy is especially recommended.

If Relapse Happens

The shock of discovering that a young woman has relapsed, after all the effort, expense, and emotional upheaval, can be as bad as or worse than dealing with the problem for the first time. One father told me he was "completely blindsided" when his son picked up again, and one mother said she was "stunned, as if I had been hit over the head with a baseball bat," when her daughter turned up high again.[3] I get it. I've been there. It can be more devastating than the first time you found out, because your expectations and hopes were raised and now they're shattered. But take a deep breath and remember: you and your daughter still have all the lessons you've worked so hard to learn, as well as new resources on your side. "A relapse," states the National Institute on Drug Abuse, "indicates a need to re-instate or adjust treatment strategy; it does not mean treatment has failed."[4] Says another eminent doctor, "It's not surprising to us that when you stop the treatment, people relapse. It doesn't mean that the treatment doesn't work, it just means that you need to continue treatment."[5]

The counselor I met with to discuss my daughter's situation at her first rehab told me gently, but firmly, that young adult addicts often use again. I nodded in agreement, but I was angry and I refused to accept it—until my daughter did use drugs again, and again. In the process, she lost her car, pawned my small amount of gold jewelry, and, most importantly, put her health in jeopardy, becoming gaunt and sick with infections and sores that refused to heal. We have to remember substance use disorder is a chronic condition, a disease that can recur just like diabetes, hypertension, and asthma can recur.

My daughter says she hated that time in her life; she couldn't get "high" anymore, but was using constantly to ward off getting "dope sick"—that is, withdrawal symptoms. She stumbled around recovery for some time after that.

For all these reasons, I urge you to have a relapse plan in place, just in case. Here are some of the elements to include in the plan:

- **Be open and honest with her**. If you suspect or know your daughter is using again, do not ignore it. Let her know you're concerned.
- **Remember your boundaries**. Let her know what you will and will not accept. For example, will you allow your daughter to continue to live at home if she picks up again? Under what conditions would she be allowed to remain at home?
- **Do not enable her**. I dislike the term "helicopter mom," but it was hard to avoid getting sucked into those whirling blades as my daughter was growing up. In the middle-class suburban subculture she grew up in, concern among parents easily slid into control, and I got used to trying to "fix" everything for my daughter while making excuses (rationalizing) that I wasn't. It was a classic mistake: not giving her enough of an opportunity to feel and process her own mistakes as a teenager.
- **Encourage her to get help**. How often I've had to remind myself that this does not mean nagging or threatening! What does help look like for your young adult? It might mean returning to a rehab facility for more treatment—some treatment centers have specific programs for those who relapse, so ask about these when you inquire. It might be a schedule of twelve-step meetings, or encouraging her to see a counselor.

The course a young person will take is up to her, with our constant encouragement and firm boundaries. My mantra during this hellish period became, "I cannot assume responsibility for my daughter's recovery." As another parent with a lot of experience put it: "Don't get sucked into the drama." She advised me to stick to the script of offering support for any effort my child would make to get better.

I remember a terrible day when Kim was about twenty and in one of her frequent periods of having moved back home. It was a beautiful summer day, and she'd slept through most of it, as usual, when she finally got up and shambled out to the backyard patio. I was doing my version of after-work relaxing, which at that time meant drinking too much coffee, smoking, and paging through a magazine. She mumbled "hey," the height of our communication then, aside from her attempts to get money from me. She was wearing pajama pants from middle school decorated with pink elephants and a ripped, not very clean T-shirt. She had lost so much weight her pants barely stayed on her hips. Her hair was unwashed and knotted, and there were sores on her face and a wound on her leg that wasn't healing.

In that moment I had a rare moment of clarity: I realized my very best efforts had led me to this: two dysfunctional physical and emotional wrecks. Then a strange new sensation came over me: I felt a weight lift off my chest.

"I can't do this anymore," I heard myself say. "I can't stand seeing you like this and I can't stand feeling like this. I'm done. I'll always help you try to get well, but I need you to quit using or leave."

Tears rolled down both our faces. Kim and I were talked and yelled out. We had made agreements; we had seen them all fall apart in the grip of her addiction. She kept trying to get better, she kept going back. And it kept getting worse. Now I had declared my end to this ghastly game. From that moment on, there was a shift in the dynamics of our relationship. Did she magically enter recovery because of my soul's cry? No, but that wasn't the point. I just wasn't going to wait around for the next dreadful phone call, the next cop car in the driveway, the next ambulance, then turn around to help her out of the mess.

This epiphany did not result in her instant sobriety. There was more to come, a lot more, and mercifully I was not to know about some of it until years later. However, now there was clear acknowledgement of the damage of addiction and of the need for her to take responsibility.

Notes on Chapter Nine

1. Shari Roan, "The 30-Day Myth," *Los Angeles Times* (November 10, 2008).

2. The Council on Accreditation of Peer Recovery Support Services (CAPRSS), www.caprss.org.

3. David Sheff, author and father of a son in recovery, speaking at an addiction forum at Odyssey House, Shrub Oak, New York, in March of 2014; and a mother of a daughter in recovery I interviewed in May, 2014.

4. National Institute on Drug Abuse (NIDA), "Seeking Drug Abuse Treatment: Know What to Ask," (last updated June 2013), www.drugabuse.gov/publications/seeking-drug-abuse-treatment-know-what-to-ask.

5. Daniel Alford, MD, Associate Professor of Medicine, Boston University School of Medicine, quoted in "Addiction Medicine: Closing the Gap Between Science and Medicine," National Center on Addiction and Substance Abuse at Columbia University (CASA), June 2012, http://www.casacolumbia.org/addiction-research/reports/addiction-medicine.

Chapter Ten

· · · · · · · ·

Be There As You Can

"Addiction teaches us many lessons. One of the most profound is that we cannot control anyone except ourselves. The lesson applies equally to recovery."[1] So writes one mother of a daughter with a substance use problem. We can, and should, benefit from such hard-won knowledge.

Keep Getting Support

Our lives have been overloaded with crises, stoking us with fear, rage, shame, and guilt. Hope and joy are frequently dashed. Dealing with the fallout from a child's addiction can leave little time or energy for other people in our lives, let alone ourselves. Children, spouses, friends, and family may be ignored and might pull away as a result, leaving us with a deeper sense of isolation and guilt. Former Senator George McGovern poignantly describes the resentment he would feel from his other children, who naturally questioned whether a father who was so involved with one daughter was still capable of truly caring for them. At times he would demonstratively distance himself from his alcoholic daughter when she needed him most in order to demonstrate to his other children that he wasn't entirely lost to their sister.[2]

What we need to ask, regardless of the circumstances, is what about *our* needs? Whether we have been caregivers, rescuers, enforcers or "just" parents, we have probably neglected our own lives. Looking back, I now see that I became obsessed with trying to get my daughter well so that my natural instincts were distorted. For example, I called her on her cell phone ten, twenty times a day when she didn't call me back. Even now, after she has been in recovery for several years, my obsession hasn't folded its tent. I still find it challenging to toe the line between being helpful and controlling—to accept that *she* has to learn to take charge of her young life. Deep down I'm terrified to let go, to accept that being present for myself doesn't mean I am abandoning my child, who is now an adult.

Our culture places tremendous importance on self-reliance. But in crisis, it is healthy to turn to others, to a community. Other people help me get clear about stepping away and following my own blurred instincts, or just offer me a cup of coffee and conversation. I need objective, informed advice to nudge me out of my habits and urge me forward again, and I especially need it when I feel that tug of resistance. At different times this has included counseling, a support group, and now the desire to give back, to do whatever I can for others going through what I went through. I have met wonderful people I would never have known if I hadn't reached out. They help me relax and laugh, and restore a healthy perspective about my role in my daughter's life.

Please consult the Appendix for lists, resources, and groups I hope will be of help to you in this journey.

The Gift of Loving Detachment

A young woman dealing with her addiction, its consequences, and its aftereffects is greatly helped by our loving detachment. When I first heard this phrase I confused it with being unsupportive, even with abandoning my child, as I watched powerlessly over her self-destruction. But in reality, loving detachment is the cultivation of healthy practical and emotional boundaries between ourselves and others.

In practicing loving detachment with my addicted daughter, I need to avoid unrealistic expectations. As someone once wonderfully put it, going into treatment to enter recovery isn't like putting a load of clothes in the washing machine. It is a complex process, and there may well be bumps along the road. Especially for a young person, impulse control and life skills must be added to the mix. Quitting using is akin to clearing the decks—it is then that the underlying issues can be addressed. Some parents want to sweep the whole experience under the rug once their daughter has gotten help. We may start to think it wasn't that bad. But recovery is like peeling away the layers of an onion—whenever I'm tempted to minimize or edit the experience of Kim's addiction, I reach into my grab bag of memories, and the reality reasserts itself: she's got work to do! Then I try to let the painful memory go. (I'm reminded of the fellowship saying: "Look at the past, but don't stare at it.") Addiction is a chronic disease and like all chronic diseases, there is no cure—but there is recovery, one day at a time.

Giving Her Choices and Respect Gives Them to You

It can seem like a paradox. A parent tries so hard to help her addicted child, to protect and sustain her. Isn't that what a good parent should do? But we learn this is not always healthy for her or for us. Just as we let our child wobble off on her bike the first time, get on a school bus, or drive a car, so we are well-advised now to let her grow her way into recovery.

As she's learning, many of us face uncomfortable but valid insights: the damaged trust between us and our child won't be rebuilt overnight. Addicts can do hurtful and careless things while in the grip of their habit. With our now-recovering child, each of us has to decide how much we're willing to trust her. For a long time, I wasn't comfortable leaving my handbag around Kim. I'd had too many bad experiences with missing money and filched credit cards. The harm from the past heals slowly.

This young adult woman who I prayed would get into recovery can be irritating at times. She procrastinates about things I think are important, and it's easy to assume she's just lazy or unmotivated. The reality is our recovering daughters are dealing with the tremendous fears that underlie and fuel alcoholism and drug addiction in the first place. Because she's in recovery, she's facing her fears and her emotions without the buffer, distraction, and/or false bravado she got from using. Those fears may include not being good, smart or pretty enough—and not measuring up to what her parents expect of her. She is more vulnerable than she'll ever let you know. I've learned to applaud my daughter for her efforts and take a deep breath when she "disappoints" me.

As I saw my behavior with Kim in a new light, I had to own up to all kinds of unspoken assumptions I had about her. I realized I'd written a script for her future that deleted the mistakes I felt my parents had made with me. In it, I also deleted the mistakes I had made as a young woman. Of course, it doesn't work that way. But even when it was clear she had become an addict in free fall, I clung desperately to my tattered script for her. It took me a while to own up to the fact that it was my script and my dreams, not Kim's. I was pouring all this energy into her—but it was really about me.

Accepting this realization hasn't been easy. But the best part has been discovering that she is writing her own script. This daughter of mine has many worthwhile dreams—some of which may seem wacky and unrealistic from my point of view, for what it's worth—but they are dreams that are *hers*. Unless they are dangerous or completely impractical, I now listen to her ideas without criticizing her or "offering suggestions." Whether she fulfills them is up to her. And while she's often impulsive, scattered, and thoughtless, she also amazes me with her accomplishments and insights. "The early years of recovery," says author Barbara Conyers, "often include continued impairment of emotional and social functioning. Healthy behavior can take years. They don't have much practice."[3] Well, neither do I with being the parent of an addict. But we parents can practice, too.

Practicing Self-Care

While Kim was numbing herself to pain and the effects of her actions, I experienced all the blows without the benefit of anesthesia and became emotionally exhausted. By taking small steps, manageable bites of pleasure, letting a few trusted people back into my life, I began to reconnect with the world. Along the way I heard a fascinating phrase: "extreme self-care." Like extreme sports? Indulging in the most expensive bubble bath I could afford? Gorging at five-star French restaurants? Standing on my head in advanced yoga classes? Well, no. . . . The point was my life had narrowed and darkened like a bad dream. The people and things I loved had been put on the shelf. I liked going to concerts, movies, plays, museums, swimming, gardening, and restaurants. But as Kim became sicker, so did I. I could be found mostly in front of the television watching reruns, eating takeout and lots of sweets. I even took up smoking after thirty years of being nicotine-free. (I've since quit, again.) I didn't want to talk to anyone. I just wanted to be numb. How was this helping?

Extreme self-care means really paying attention to your own needs. My counselor advised me that to do this, I needed to set modest goals for myself and periodically remind myself I wasn't being a "bad mother" by taking care of myself. So I made a list. I called the people in my life I'd been neglecting, starting with my son, who understandably felt abandoned by me, as well as angry at his sister, then other family members and friends. I planned simple outings, refocused on my work, ate better, and exercised some. I recharged my spiritual batteries, which included regular prayer and meditation. When I do this, my thoughts slow down, and I have more clarity about whatever is going on.

Letting Go of Shame and Blame

Taking care of myself meant I needed to forgive myself before I could forgive my daughter. I had made many mistakes with her, but I hadn't put the drink in her hand or the needle in her arm. Those were the decisions of her active addiction.

Remember:

You did not cause it. You can't change the past, but you *can* focus on the present. Let go of your guilt. You are at a new place and you will do things differently.

You cannot control it. If an addicted person wants to get drugs, she'll find them. The best you can do is model a healthy lifestyle, offer her loving suggestions and good boundaries. It is possible to force someone to get treatment, but that doesn't mean she'll accept the gift of long-term recovery. Acceptance that there is a lot we as parents can do, but only so much, can give us a more peaceful state of mind.

You cannot cure it. Again, the addict will only be helped when she accepts responsibility and takes steps to change her own life.

Today, Kim and I are leading our own lives and we enjoy the time we spend together. What a relief! Yes, there's hope! Living comfortably without alcohol or other drugs is a reality for millions of people who once were addicted. Sometimes it just "clicks," but more often, there's a kind of emotional dance in recovery: Two steps forward, one step back, slide, and forward again. Sometimes an addicted child does not get well, and as a leading expert in the field advises, "All the evidence-based treatments and loving support systems in the world don't seem to touch them. . . . If you've done your best, and can't do any more, we hope that you can go on treating yourself kindly and go forward with the care and support in your life that you deserve."[4]

It feels good when I focus on what makes me happy and fulfilled, rather than on what I don't have in my life. It is a relief to know I am not responsible for my daughter's life—she is. It is good to know there is support freely available to me, that I am far from being alone in dealing with a young adult daughter in recovery. It is a daunting fact that drug and alcohol abuse by young people has been identified as our nation's number one health problem. With the right tools, we all stand a good chance of healing.

Informed, Healthy Choices

Over the last two decades both lay people and professionals in the field of addiction treatment have come to recognize how both normal functioning and the experience of disease—including substance use disorder—differ between the genders. The implications have been life-changing for women and men alike and will continue to be so as the research advances. It is my hope that this information will help you deal with a female child suffering from substance use disorder.

Moving from addiction to recovery is a tough journey, but it is also exhilarating and liberating. No one needs do it alone or without support. From my own experience and from thousands of recovering people I've heard speak candidly about their experiences, I know women and men make tremendous progress with the issues that were underlying and driving their addiction. When we face the reality of a beloved child's chronic disease of addiction, everything we as parents do to lovingly and firmly offer healthy choices as alternatives to her self-destruction increases her chances of recovery and ours of accepting reality.

As we offer our daughters healthy choices, let's not forget to offer them to ourselves!

I wish you serenity on your journey.

Notes on Chapter Ten

1. Barbara Conyers, *Everything Changes: Help For Families of Newly Recovering Addicts* (Center City, MN: Hazelden, 2009), 20.

2. George McGovern, *Terry: My Daughter's Life-and-Death Struggle with Alcoholism* (New York: Villard Books, 1995), 194.

3. Conyers, *Everything Changes*, 117.

4. Jeffrey Foote, Carrie Wilkens, and Nicole Kosanke, with Stephanie Higgs, *Beyond Addiction: How Science and Kindness Help People Change* (New York: Scribner, 2014), 277.

Chapter Eleven
. . . .

Just Say Yes: What's New
and What You Can Do

We in America are at a crossroads in terms of how we think about, educate people, and treat substance use, and many valiant efforts are being made. One example is the shift from criminalizing those who suffer from addiction to focusing on getting them into treatment. Another is the legal and advocacy efforts to rein in the over-prescribing of opioids. For instance, Physicians for Responsible Opioid Prescribing (SupportProp. org) work to educate physicians and to implement laws to limit the amount of opioids prescribed. Also, the Medicine Abuse Project at The Partnership for Drug-Free Kids (DrugFree.org) offers parents a pledge to help end medicine abuse by learning more, safeguarding medicine, and talking with the teens in our lives.

Some states have passed bills that would ban synthetic (designer) drugs; require education for doctors who prescribe opioids; make prescription monitoring programs mandatory to stop "doctor shopping"; implement Good Samaritan laws that protect those who call the police during an overdose even if they were also using illegal drugs; and expand the use of the drug overdose antidote "naloxone," known as Narcan, which immediately cancels the effects of an overdose. A nasal spray formulation has been introduced for easier use in some communities.

On the other hand, powerful lobbies thwart other efforts. Over strong protests by the majority of the FDA's own advisory panel, in 2014 the FDA approved a powerful new, non-tamper-proof opioid painkiller called Zohydro ER. Zohydro is a long-acting form of hydrocodone, the first opioid not to contain acetaminophen, which can cause liver damage if used frequently. But Zohydro is said to be five to ten times more powerful than Vicodin. A note of caution: though this book is about addiction in young women, an increasing number of older Americans who are prescribed opioid painkillers have become addicted. It is worth noting again that the use of opioids to treat pain over a lengthy period has been disputed as an effective strategy, not to mention the drug dependence that can often result. Meanwhile, the alcohol industry remains powerfully entrenched.

Thankfully, grassroots efforts to combat the epidemic of addiction to drugs and alcohol is growing exponentially among young people in recovery, parents of addicted children, research scientists, and treatment professionals. For young women and men, there are more and more effective tools for recovery.

Some parents who have lived with an addicted child are relieved to return to a life free from the ongoing crisis of the disorder and its cares. Others feel the need to get involved in furthering the movement toward better treatment, better policies, greater awareness of and access to help. I invite you to review your own experience. When you realized your daughter had a problem, did you feel the schools, doctors, and therapists you turned to really helped? If you looked for treatment, was that experience clearly explained to you and worth the investment? Evidently, a lot of us have unhelpful and negative experiences. Some realize a lot of doctors don't know that much about preventing, identifying, or treating this epidemic.[1] And many of us agree with the statement that "addiction medicine is at least forty years behind where it could and should be."[2]

There are hardworking individuals and organizations seeking to improve the standards of education for physicians about the complexity of addiction, the regulations and standards of the treatment industry, the needs for tailored approaches for particular genders, ages, and ethnicities . . . and the list goes on. Some parent groups are stepping into the gap and are taking it upon themselves to provide effective prevention education to elementary schools on up.

At a recent forum for parents about drug prevention and use, author David Sheff, father of a son now in recovery, dug into this topic. Scare tactics and "just say no" have not proven to be effective deterrents for our kids. Stress, both externally and internally imposed, is known to be a key factor in many young people's decision to try drugs and alcohol. But what, Sheff asked, are our children's schools doing to teach kids to be resilient, to gain insight into what causes them stress and how to deal with it? Are schools providing evidence-based programs of prevention, intervention, and help? From my experience as an active parent, the answer is "not much." From the time my daughter was in her second semester as a freshman until she miraculously managed to graduate from high school, I was called in to meet with teachers, advisors, and the principal. While they were all concerned about Kim's worsening grades and absenteeism, the topic of her possible drug use didn't come up until she went to an alternative senior year program that had little bureaucracy or face-saving to worry about. Kim's classmates were typical suburban kids. Most of them were on track and pushed to be high achievers. But a good number of them were obviously troubled. It was a poorly kept secret that some kids brought alcohol to classes in water bottles and that others traded marijuana and pills around the campus. Yet the parents' organization continued to concern itself with the familiar PTA bake-sale stuff, while this or that student would disappear for a month or three—off to rehab. There were the occasional overdoses and, of course, the tragic car crashes. But it was treated like business as usual.

Now at last there is strong advocacy for a curriculum that teaches emotion-focused, healthy alternatives to dealing with stress, along with a solidly-researched curriculum of drug education for the ever-growing number of our children who are turning to substances.

In communities across the land, we see average folks who are stunned and frightened by their children's substance use and sometimes, tragically, by their overdoses. In the county I live in, after two sets of parents lost wonderful sons to opiate addiction despite all their best efforts to help them, they started an organization called "Drug Crisis in our Backyard."

It reaches out to parents, schools, law enforcement, state legislators, and kids through forums, support groups, and lobbying efforts, and they are making a real impact. Your community may have, or need, a similar group.

Loving Ourselves Is the Best Medicine

When Kim was in her active addiction, I was not a normal person. And today I am not the same person I was before she became addicted. Despite the pain and chaos that only another parent of an addicted child can understand, I believe I am more empathetic and more realistic today. I was always steeling myself for the next crisis that was sure to ambush me anyway. My obsession with her life was choking me.

When Kim had put together a year in recovery (or so I thought) she came "home" to visit. Kim had moved across the country, where I thought she was going to twelve-step meetings, classes at a community college, and a part-time job. But within hours of her arrival at home, she confessed, sobbing, that she had used some heroin she'd picked up at the local Dunkin' Donuts. The English have an expression: "gobsmacked." And that is how I felt. How could this have happened? But it was simple enough. Slowly during that year, she'd drifted away from her support system, and had stopped telling people in her recovery group about how she was feeling. Soon, she was no longer going to classes, though she did hang on to her job. She was back to "partying," drinking and smoking pot, while managing to stay away from opioids. Over that year, she began to fantasize about getting high on heroin just one more time. But after she used, Kim became terrified and immediately "ratted herself out," as she put it. "Mom," she was to tell me later, "you were awesome the way you handled it. You listened to me and processed the whole thing in about fifteen minutes. First, you said you were angry and disappointed in me, that you understood about the disease but you could not have me stay in the house using. That I had to get rid of anything else I'd hidden. That you'd support me emotionally and financially to get into recovery and that I should go to a [twelve-step] meeting right away. If not, I was on my own."

Was I "awesome"? Hardly, though I'm glad she thought so. I was crushed, devastated. We'd had the "talk," and I'd laid down my bottom line a year before, yet here we were again. However, I had been continuing to "work on myself" during that time and something had again shifted within me—there was a new clarity. I knew I couldn't do the work she needed to do for herself; I knew I had to take care of myself. I couldn't "save" her anymore. And I've come to understand taking care of myself doesn't mean being selfish or indifferent to the sufferings of others (above all, my children's). Rather, it's a kind of enlightened self-interest. It invites in light and air where darkness and fear have reigned for so long. I invite you, if you haven't done so already, to practice loving detachment from trying to fix a sick daughter and instead to help her reach for good choices.

My daughter has been in recovery since that last "experiment." It is one day at a time. She says what helped her most the last time she used drugs was my firmness and her own burning need to take responsibility. *Really?* My rule-busting girl said that? But it makes real sense: She had experienced many of the personally satisfying benefits of recovery. And to be held accountable promotes self-respect. It gives a beaten-down person the dignity of having choices. Helping a young woman see she has choices, and that you expect and know that she can make them, is not enabling but empowering.

I've talked a lot about the importance of taking care of ourselves in the midst of the storm of addiction in our beloved children. It may feel like betrayal to let go, but here's a powerful nudge: To effectively help others, we have got to help ourselves. If I'm a basket case, I can't be effective for my child. Going down the rabbit hole with her won't help her, and it won't help you and your other loved ones. Science and treatment can take us but only so far. Love can take us farther. But in the end, the addicted person has to become involved in her own recovery.

Since I gave up trying to have the power to give her recovery, it hasn't always been a smooth ride for Kim and me. Getting into recovery means facing what twelve-step fellowships call the "wreckage of our past." For a young woman in recovery that includes confronting deep insecurities, the traumatic experiences she may have had, and learning to be responsible and make healthy decisions—all the while surrounded by other young people who may be indulging in casual or serious drug or alcohol use. But Kim has a support system and a good sponsor, a woman with more years in recovery who can give counsel from her own experience. Kim is awake to her life now, and she's doing many of the things she fantasized about while she was using. As for me, I continue to work on myself. I know I am a soft touch (I learned this from my mother). I have, after years of recovery, no trouble accepting I am an addict, but as a mother, I still at times resist the reality that my child is an addict, that she has a chronic illness that can be arrested but not cured. I am also reassured by knowing there are supportive and loving people who are willing to help me continue to change and grow. Because loving ourselves helps us love our children in healthy ways, and this gives them and us the best hope for a good, productive life.

Notes on Chapter Eleven

1. See National Center on Addiction and Substance Abuse at Columbia University (CASA), "Missed Opportunity: A National Survey of Primary Care Physicians and Patients on Substance Abuse" (April 2000).

2. David Sheff, *Clean: Overcoming Addiction and Ending America's Greatest Tragedy* (New York: Houghton Mifflin Harcourt, 2013), 275.

Resources

Twelve-Step Resources for Parents and Loved Ones of Substance Users

Al-Anon
Nationwide, free support to family and friends of alcoholics.
Alateen is for family members in their teens.
www.al-anon.org
www.al-anon.alateen.org

Nar-Anon
Nationwide, free support to family and friends of substance
abusers. Literature includes a helpful checklist for members.
Narateen is for family members in their teens.
www.nar-anon.org

Co-Dependents Anonymous (CoDA)
A twelve-step program that supports recovery of people in
codependent relationships. (Codependency is popularly defined
as an addiction to having a supportive role in a relationship. Also,
the codependent person facilitates the behavior of the one who is
dependent on a substance or process.)
www.coda.org

Families Anonymous
Supports parents of alcoholics and addicts.
www.familiesanonymous.org

Adult Children of Alcoholics (ACoA)
A twelve-step program that supports recovery of those raised in alcoholic or otherwise dysfunctional households. www.adultchildren.org.

Other Twelve-Step Resources

Alcoholics Anonymous online
www.e-aa.org

Narcotics Anonymous online
www.na-recovery.org

Recovery-Related Blogs and Websites

The Addict's Mom
A blog that connects mothers of addicts to share their experiences. The site offers many resources. www.addictsmom.com

Parent Pathway
www.parentpathway.com/blog

Faces and Voices of Recovery
www.facesandvoicesofrecovery.org

The Fix
www.thefix.com

In the Rooms
www.intherooms.com

Renew: Your Addiction and Recovery Source
www.reneweveryday.com

Suboxone Talk Zone
Blog addresses the pros and cons of this medication. www.suboxonetalkzone.com

Young People in Recovery
www.youngpeopleinrecovery.org

Public and Private Organizations/Resources

Communities That Care (CTC)
A coalition-based community system that uses a public health
approach to prevent youth problem behaviors.
www.communitiesthatcare.net

The Council on Alcohol and Drug Abuse
www.dallascouncil.org

Intervention Services for Youth: Safe Interventions
Specializes in adolescent transportation services and crisis
intervention.
www.safeinterventions.com

MADD (Mothers Against Drunk Driving)
Has a campaign called "Power of Parents."
www.madd.org/powerofparents

Mediate.com
Serves as a bridge between professionals offering mediation services
and people needing mediation services.
www.mediate.com

National Domestic Violence Hotline
1-800-799-7233
www.ndvh.org

National Institute on Drug Abuse (NIDA)
www.drugabuse.gov

Parents Helpline
A nationwide support for parents and other caregivers who want to talk to someone about their child's drug use and drinking. English and Spanish.
1-855-378-4373

The Parent Toolkit
A helpful guide for concerned parents from first graders on up.
www.theparenttoolkit.org

Partnership for Drug-Free Kids
Extensive resources for parents.
www.drugfree.org

Posttraumatic Stress Disorder Alliance
1-877-507-7873
www.ptsdalliance.org

Psychology Today's Therapy Directory
Provides a comprehensive directory of therapists, psychiatrists, and treatment facilities near you.
www.psychologytoday.com

Recovery Happens Counseling Services
Based in California, the services include a great deal of information for parents, including webinars, and recommendations for treatment centers for adolescents.
www.recoveryhappens.com

Shatterproof
An organization "committed to ending the suffering of our loved ones and protecting our children from addiction's grip." Seeks to become a national entity to coordinate best practices in all aspects of addiction, including specific prevention and

treatment programming; working with the medical profession; and community prevention programs. Resources for parents. www.shatterproof.org

Vital Intervention Professionals (VIP)
www.viprecovery.com

Selected List of Gender-Separate Treatment Facilities

When I first began to research gender-specific facilities for women several years ago, I discovered there was no central data center for such listings. In fact, one employee at a large government agency expressed surprise that women-specific treatment facilities even existed. The list below, culled from many resources, is by no means exhaustive, and inclusion is not intended as an endorsement, but rather as a guide for you. For additional listings visit Women.InterventionAmerica.org.

Women-Only Facilities

Awakenings at Serenity Hill, Hemet, California
Rehabilitation, dual-diagnosis, transitional and sober living.
1-888-629-3330

Brookhaven Retreat, outside of Knoxville, Tennessee
"Life Realignment Program," also called "Poncho." Includes treatment also for self-injury, borderline personality disorder, and emotional eating. Not based on the Twelve Steps.
www.brookhavenretreat.com

Casa de las Amigas, Pasadena, California
Includes residential, outpatient, and sober living facilities.
www.casadelasamigas.org

Clearview Women's Center, Venice, California
Treats addiction and women's psychiatric issues, including borderline personality disorder.
www.clearviewwomenscenter.com

Hannah's House by Origins Recovery Centers,
South Padre Island, Texas
Treats relapsing, dual-diagnosed women in a "boutique" program.
www.originsrecovery.com

Harmony Place Treatment, Los Angeles, California
Treats addiction, also acute dual diagnosis, in a high-end facility.
www.harmonyplace.com

The Haven, Tucson, Arizona
Serves homeless and near-homeless women; includes facilities for
young children. Has "Native Ways" program for Native Americans.
www.thehaventucson.org

Liberty Place Recovery Center for Women, Richmond, Kentucky
For homeless women eighteen and older. Free to area residents.
www.foothillscap.org

New Directions for Women, Newport Beach, California
Treatment for chemical dependency for women age eighteen and
above, pregnant women, and women with dependent children.
www.newdirectionsforwomen.org

Nexus Recovery Center, Dallas, Texas
For adult women, adolescent girls ages thirteen to seventeen.
Includes pregnant women or those with children.
www.nexusrecovery.org

New Hope Manor, Barryville, New York
For adolescents, adults, pregnant women, women with infants, and
criminal-justice clients. Offers accredited college, high school, and
GED classes.
www.newhopemanor.org

The Orchid Recovery Center, West Palm Beach, Florida
See also page 91.
www.orchidrecoverycenter.com

Pine Grove Women's Center, Hattiesburg, Mississippi
Has separate programs for eating disorders, chemical dependency,
and dual addiction.
www.pinegrovetreatment.com

Recovery Center for Women of the Palm Beaches, Palm Beach, Florida
Part of the Behavioral Health of the Palm Beaches. Includes many
specialties related to women's issues and tiered programs.
www.rehabcenterforwomen.org

Residence XII, Kirkland, Washington
Established in 1981. Women-centered treatment and family
programs.
www.residencexii.org

The Rose, Newport Beach, California
Addiction treatment for women eighteen to seventy and older.
Provides access to college program. A program of Sober Living by
the Sea Treatment Centers.
www.therose.crchealth.com

Safe Harbor Treatment Center for Women, Los Angeles
A ninety-day program with sober living facility for aftercare.
www.safeharborhouse.com

Seaside Center for Women, Palm Beach, Florida
Upscale and run by the Behavioral Health of the Palm Beaches.
www.rehabcenterforwomen.org

Susan B. Anthony Recovery Center, Fort Lauderdale, Florida
Accepts addicted mothers with children.
www.susanbanthonycenter.org

Timberline Knolls, Lemont, Illinois
For adolescents twelve and older and adult women. Also treats a range of eating disorders and self-injury. Includes The Academy: an accredited, licensed high school that includes Advanced Placement classes, ACT/SAT prep, and tutoring. Also offers an optional individualized Christian Treatment program.
www.timberlineknolls.com

Transformations by the Gulf, St. Pete Beach, Florida
Outpatient; with residential housing if needed. Gender-separate, eighteen and over. As well as substance abuse, specializes in process addictions, such as cutting, eating disorders, gambling, etc.
www.transformationsbythegulf.com

Women's Recovery Association, Burlingame, California
Inpatient programs, including residential for women, pregnant women (with Perinatal Treatment), mothers with children, and a specific program for young women eighteen to twenty-four.
www.womensrecovery.org

Selection of Facilities for Both Genders that Offer Separate Programs for Women and Men

Balboa Horizons, Newport Beach, California
www.balboahorizons.com

Benchmark Recovery Center, Austin, Texas
www.benchmarkcenter.com

Betty Ford Center, Rancho Mirage, California
A Part of the Hazelden Betty Ford Foundation
See also page 96.
www.bettyfordcenter.org

Caron Centers, Wernersville, Pennsylvania (main campus)
See also page 93.
www.caron.org

Creative Care, Malibu, California
Specializes in dual diagnosis treatment. Also addresses eating disorders, self-harm, sex addiction, gambling, relationship addictions, and obsessive-compulsive disorder.
www.creativecareinc.com

Hanley Center at Origins, Center for Women's Recovery, West Palm Beach, Florida
An Origins Recovery Center
For ages eighteen to forty-six. Includes a family program and alumni aftercare for two years.
www.originsrecovery.com

Progress Valley Women's Program, Richfield, Minnesota
Offers sober housing in aftercare.
(Men's program, Minneapolis, Minnesota)
www.progressvalley.org

The Ranch in Tennessee, Nunnelly, Tennessee
Separate facilities for women and men ages eighteen and older. Life skills oriented. Includes Native American healing rituals (sweat lodge, medicine wheel, Toltec wisdom), as well as twelve-step approach.
www.recoveryranch.com

Gender-Separate Facilities for Adolescents and Young Adults
Betty Ford Center, Rancho Mirage, California
(See page 144)
www.bettyfordcenter.org

Caron Treatment Center, Wernersville, Pennsylvania (main campus)
(See page 144)
www.caron.org

Hazelden Center, Youth and Families Campus, Medicine Lake,
Plymouth, Minnesota
(See page 94)
www.hazelden.org

Inspirations, Fort Lauderdale, Florida
For youth aged fourteen to eighteen. Residential treatment,
including educational program and full treatment facilities.
www.inspirationsyouth.com

New Hope Manor, Barryville, New York
(See page 142)
www.newhopemanor.org

Newport Academy, Newport Beach, California
www.newportacademy.com

Phoenix House Academy of Westchester, Shrub Oak, New York
Treats adolescent boys and girls for addiction, and offers high
school accredited education, including vocational curricula.
Accepts Medicaid.
www.phoenixhouse.org

Sweetwater Adolescent Girls Treatment Program
At Cottonwood Tucson, Tucson, Arizona
For ages thirteen to seventeen. Ninety-day program with a
scholastic component. Treats addiction, self-harm, trauma, eating
disorders, ADD, mental disorders, and more.
www.cottonwooddetucson.com

Timberline Knolls, Lemont, Illinois
For adolescent women aged twelve and above.
(See page 144)
www.timberlineknolls.com

Association of Recovery Schools
Lists high schools and colleges that host programs for young people after treatment.
www.recoveryschools.org

Facilities for Women with Children

Austin Recovery, Austin, Texas
Offers men's and women's programs, including for women with young children.
www.austinrecovery.org

Jefferson University Hospital, Maternal Addiction Treatment Education and Research (MATER) Program, Philadelphia, Pennsylvania
Offers treatment for substance-abusing pregnant and parenting women and their children, both outpatient and residential.
www.jefferson.edu/university/jmc/departments/pediatrics/mother/contact.html

Magnolia Women's Recovery Program, Hayward, California
Serves pregnant and postpartum women and women with children from birth through age five.
www.magnoliarecovery.org

Marin Services for Women, Greenbrae, California
Includes women with children aged six and under.
1-415-924-5995

Miriam's House, The Promises Foundation, Culver City, California
A one-year, four-phase program for women with dependent children.
www.promisesfoundation.org

New Directions for Women, Newport Beach, California
See also page 142.
www.newdirectionsforwomen.org

New Hope Manor, Barryville, New York
See also page 142.
www.newhopemanor.org

Rural Women's Recovery Program, Athens, Ohio
Serves adult women, including with children ages five and under.
www.hrs.org

Susan B. Anthony Recovery Center, Fort Lauderdale, Florida
Specializes in addicted women with dependent children.
www.susanbanthonycenter.org

Women-Only Facilities that Address Borderline Personality Issues
Borderline personality disorder typically involves a great degree of instability in mood and black/white thinking (splitting), such as switching between extremes in thinking. For example: everything is great or everything is terrible.

Brookhaven Retreat, Knoxville, Tennessee
(See page 141)
www.brookhavenretreat.com

Clearview Women's Center, Venice, California
(See page 141)
www.clearviewwomenscenter.com

Women-Only Facilities that Address Process Addictions, Including Self-Harm (Cutting), Eating Disorders, and Gambling
Process addictions are behavioral addictions that do not rely on drugs.

Brookhaven Retreat, Knoxville, Tennessee
(See page 141)
www.brookhavenretreat.com

Creative Care, Malibu, California
(See page 145)
www.creativecareinc.com

Pine Grove Women's Center, Hattiesburg, Mississippi
(See page 143)
www.pinegrovetreatment.com

Timberline Knolls, Lemont, Illinois
(See page 144)
www.timberlineknolls.com

Transformations by the Gulf, St. Pete Beach, Florida
(See page 144)
www.transformationsbythegulf.com

The Victorian Treatment Center, Newport Beach, California.
Specializes in women with eating disorders. A part of Sober Living
by the Sea.
www.soberliving.com

Help for the Whole Family

Many treatment centers offer a Parent Day or Weekend, involving seminars
and workshops. Several with established programs are listed below.

The Betty Ford Center, Rancho Mirage, California
(See page 96)
www.bettyfordcenter.org

Caron Center, Wernersville, Pennsylvania (main campus)
(See page 93)
www.caron.org

Hazelden Family Program Services
(See page 94)
www.hazelden.org

For Lesbian and Bisexual Women with Addiction

Pride Institute
800-54-PRIDE (77433)
www.pride-institute.com

Sober Recovery
A lot of information about lesbian and gay recovery centers and support organizations for LGBT substance-abusers and their families.
www.soberrecovery.com/links/gayandlesbianresources.html

Gays and Lesbians in Alcoholics Anonymous (GaL-AA)
Maintains twelve-step meeting lists around the country for LGBT members.
www.gal-aa.org

Other Resources to Find Treatment Sites

The Substance Abuse and Mental Health Services Administration of the United States Department of Health and Human Services (SAMHSA) lists about 11,000 treatment sites throughout the country. SAMHSA's National Registry for Evidence-Based Practices and Programs lists mental health and substance abuse facilities that have been reviewed and rated for implementation of such practices and programs, although it does not separate out gender-specific facilities.
1-800-662-4357
www.samhsa.gov
www.findtreatment.samhsa.gov
www.nrepp.samhsa.gov

Drug Rehab and Alcohol Rehab Services Treatment Referrals and Resources
www.drugandalcoholrehab.net

Choose Help
www.choosehelp.com

Addiction Resource Guide
www.addictionresourceguide.com

Treatment Solutions Network
www.treatmentsolutionsnetwork.com

Resources to Help Find a Child Who has Run Away from Treatment

Child Find of America: 1-845-883-6060
National Runaway Safeline: 1-800-786-2929 (24/7)
Find Your Missing Child: www.findyourmissingchild.org

Suggested Reading

While no other book addresses the specific, global needs of women and young women in recovery for their loved ones, following are some of the most helpful publications on experiences shared by families and friends who love an addict.

For Parents and Families of Young Women Substance Users

Conyers, Beverly. *Addict in the Family: Stories of Loss, Hope, and Recovery*, Center City, MN: Hazelden, 2003.

Conyers, Beverly. *Everything Changes: Help for Families of Newly Recovering Addicts*, Center City, MN: Hazelden, 2009.

Fletcher, Anne M. *Inside Rehab: The Surprising Truth About Addiction Treatment—and How to Get Help That Works*. New York: Penguin, 2013.

Foote, Jeffrey, Carrie Wilkens, Nicole Kosanke, with Stephanie Higgs, *Beyond Addiction: How Science and Kindness Help People Change*. New York: Scribner, 2014.

Meyers, Robert J., and Brenda L. Wolfe. *Get Your Loved One Sober: Alternatives to Nagging, Pleading, and Threatening*. Center City, MN: Hazelden, 2004.

Schaefer, Dick. *Choices & Consequences: What to Do When a Teenager Uses Alcohol/Drugs*. Center City, MN: Hazelden, 1998.

Sheff, David. *Clean: Overcoming Addiction and Ending America's Greatest Tragedy*. New York: Houghton Mifflin Harcourt, 2014.

Turrisi, Rob. *A Parent Handbook for Talking with College Students About Alcohol: A Compilation of Information from Parents, Students, and The Scientific Community*. Tufts University, 2010, www.ase.tufts.edu/healthed/documents/parentHandbook.pdf.

Books on Women and Addiction and Growth to Adulthood

Brady, Kathleen T., Sudie E. Back, and Shelly F. Greenfield, eds. *Women & Addiction: A Comprehensive Handbook*. New York: The Guilford Press, 2009.

Briggs, Cynthia A. and Jennifer L. Pepperell. *Women, Girls, and Addiction: Celebrating the Feminine in Counseling Treatment and Recovery*. New York and London: Routledge, 2009.

Brown, Stephanie. *A Place Called Self: Women, Sobriety, and Radical Transformation*. Center City, MN: Hazelden, 2004.

The National Center on Addiction and Substance Abuse (CASA) at Columbia University. *Women under the Influence*. Baltimore, MD: Johns Hopkins University Press, 2005.

Covington, Stephanie S. *Beyond Trauma: A Healing Journey for Women Workbook*. Center City, MN: Hazelden, 2003.

Covington, Stephanie S. *Helping Women Recover, Package: A Program for Treating Addiction*. San Francisco: Jossey-Bass, 2008.

Egger, Katharina S. and Leonie H. Moser, eds. *Women and Addictions: New Research*. New York: Nova Science Publishers Inc., 2009.

Jersild, Devon. *Happy Hours: Alcohol in a Woman's Life*. New York: Harper Perennial, 2002.

Johnston, Ann Dowsett. *Drink: The Intimate Relationship Between Women and Alcohol*. New York: HarperCollins, 2013.

Legato, Marianne J., ed. *Principles of Gender-Specific Medicine*. 2nd ed. London, Burlington, MA, San Diego, CA: Academic Press, 2010.

Nolen-Hoeksema, Susan. *Eating, Drinking, Overthinking: The Toxic Triangle of Food, Alcohol, and Depression*. New York: Henry Holt, 2006.

Pipher, Mary. *Reviving Ophelia*. New York: Riverhead Books, 2003.

Snyderman Nancy L. and Peg Streep. *Girl in the Mirror: Mothers and Daughters in the Years of Adolescence*. New York: Hyperion, 2003.

Straussner, Shulamith Lala Ashenberg and Stephanie Brown, eds. *The Handbook of Addiction Treatment for Women: Theory and Practice*. San Francisco: Jossey-Bass, 2002.

Accounts of Young and Adult Women

Allen, Chaney. *I'm Black and I'm Sober: The Timeless Story of a Woman's Journey Back to Sanity.* Center City, MN: Hazelden, 1995.

Cheever, Susan. *Note Found in a Bottle: My Life as a Drinker, a Memoir.* New York: Washington Square Press, 2000.

Ford, Betty. *Healing and Hope: Six Women from the Betty Ford Center Share Their Powerful Journeys of Addiction and Recovery.* New York: Penguin, 2003.

Hooks, Bell. *Sisters of the Yam: Black Women and Self-Recovery.* Cambridge, MA: South End Press, 1993.

Karr, Mary. *Lit: a Memoir.* New York: Harper Perennial, 2010.

Knapp, Caroline. *Drinking: A Love Story.* New York: Dial Press, 1997.

Lamott, Anne. *Imperfect Birds: A Novel.* New York: Riverhead Trade, 2011.

McGovern, George. *Terry: My Daughter's Life-and-Death Struggle with Alcoholism.* New York: Villard Books, 1995.

Storm, Jennifer. *Blackout Girl: Growing Up and Drying Out in America.* Center City, MN: Hazelden, 2008.

Zailckas, Koren. *Smashed: Story of a Drunken Girlhood.* New York: Penguin, 2006.

About Young and Adult Men

Kindlon, Dan, and Michael Thompson. *Raising Cain: Protecting the Emotional Life of Boys.* New York: Ballantine, 1999.

Sax, Leonard. *Why Gender Matters: What Parents and Teachers Need to Know about the Emerging Science of Sex Differences.* New York: Doubleday, 2005.

Sheff, David. *Beautiful Boy: A Father's Journey Through His Son's Addiction.* New York: Mariner Books, 2009.

Books for Women in Twelve-Step Recovery Programs

Covington, Stephanie. *A Woman's Way Through the Twelve Steps.* Center City, MN: Hazelden, 1994.

D., Lisa, ed. *Stepping Stones to Recovery For Young People: Experience the Miracle of 12 Step Recovery.* Center City, MN: Hazelden, 1991.

Iliff, Brenda. *A Woman's Guide to Recovery.* Center City, MN: Hazelden, 2008.